PRAISE FO

AFTERSH

"Dr. Utter's book, *Aftershock: How Past Events Shake Up Your Life Today*, is the beginning of therapy for everyone. On completion of the book, you realize that everyone would benefit from talking to a mental health professional, especially one who is as insightful and able to read in between the lines of your thoughts like Dr. Utter. She lays out the groundwork from the beginning of the trauma, then takes you on a step-by-step experience of how to address it. At the end of each chapter, a brief "Let's Review" section pinpoints the important issues discussed. Dr. Utter's humor and self-acknowledgement that she too benefits from therapy puts a person, even the most reluctant, at ease in understanding how to seek help and comfort. From the beginning, her personal stories are intertwined to explain how our psyches work. She then breaks it down into humorous examples for better understanding. At times, the 'lol' written on the pages really turned into 'laugh out loud' for me. I truly can say that I could not put this book down until finished and then wanted more!"

—Jan Widerman, DO, FACOP, FAAP,
FAOAAM, FASAM

"After reading *Aftershock,* I felt more at ease with myself knowing that people from all walks of life have experienced a life event that was traumatic for them. I got an educational, and hilarious, outlook on trauma and how it is different for everyone. I liked that there were personal stories shared in the book and was able to connect to them. In my opinion, learning while being able to relate and laugh is amazing. It is worth the read because once you pick it up, you'll go through all emotions and not want to put it down until it's finished. It'll leave you wanting more!"

—**Brittany Lee,** college student

AFTERSHOCK

AFTERSHOCK

How Past Events
Shake Up Your Life Today

Geri-Lynn Utter, PsyD

Health Communications, Inc.
Boca Raton, Florida

www.hcibooks.com

Author's note: While the events and details depicted in this work are true, I have disguised some patients and certain other individuals to protect their privacy.

Library of Congress Cataloging-in-Publication Data
is available through the Library of Congress

ISBN-13: 978-07573-2490-1(Paperback)
ISBN-10: 0-7573-2490-8 (Paperback)
ISBN-13: 978-0-7573-2491-8 (ePub)
ISBN-10: 0-7573-2491-6 (ePub)

Publisher: Health Communications, Inc.
      301 Crawford Boulevard, Suite 200
      Boca Raton, FL 33432–3762

Cover design by Erica Ash
Interior design and typesetting by Larissa Hise Henoch

For my dad:
Every time I doubt myself, I hear your words:
"Kid, you can do anything you put your mind to."
Thanks for always believing in me, Dad.

CONTENTS

INTRODUCTION

WHAT IS "AFTERSHOCK"?

During stressful events, even those that may seem common-place at the time, such as weddings ("'Till death . . . "?) or starting a new job ("Who are these people?"), we often suppress emotions that might render us unable to manage a situation effectively—that is, we just deal with it so we won't screw it up. The effects of trauma-related suppressed emotions can sneak up on us months after the initial trauma occurred in ways we might not recognize. Yes, it is annoying and stressful as hell. Yet, most of us will not understand why we are experiencing mental health issues when the most obvious danger has passed. No, you're not crazy. You're experiencing aftershock.

Bear with me for a moment while I get clinical. Some of this you likely know already, but here are the basics.

The most unsettling and dangerous events that humans experience can cause an emotional response, which we call psychological trauma. But not all trauma is alike; from the horrors of war to the emotional stress of seemingly mundane events in everyday life, trauma comes in infinite levels of severity.

Trauma comes in infinite levels of severity.

Further, our emotional response to trauma is not always recognized during the event. Humans often suppress their emotions during stressful times in order to deal with the situation at hand. That is, we can't just fall apart emotionally, or everything would go to hell.

These suppressed emotions do not always disappear entirely; more often, they reemerge later, creating emotional havoc. Post-traumatic stress disorder (PTSD) is the most widely recognized form of this delayed response. It is most often diagnosed in returning war veterans and others who've survived intensely traumatic events.

But just as there are many levels of trauma-inducing situations, there are numerous, less recognized levels of post-traumatic stress that may occur after less earthshaking events. I call this phenomenon aftershock.

A "subclinical" level of the more-familiar PTSD, aftershock may underlie your present emotional stress, a delayed emotional response to life's most challenging times. In short, you may find yourself emotionally out of sorts today from something that caused you significant stress in the recent past—without realizing the cause.

I will teach you about psychological trauma, what it is, and what causes it. Then you'll learn more about aftershock and how life's stressors may have put you into the center of an aftershock storm. You'll also learn how to recognize and deal with your own stress responses.

No, you're not crazy; at least you're not crazier than the rest of us. But if you're reeling from an aftershock event like so many of us, I'm here to help.

CHAPTER ONE

Aftershock: What Is Trauma and How Does It Happen?

I WANT TO HELP YOU understand how highly stressful events can wreak havoc on your mental health, how the mental trauma they cause can lead to aftershock, and how to recognize aftershock when it insidiously shakes up your world.

We'll start with the basics. There are three major types of trauma: chronic, complex, and acute. You'll learn what defines each. I will use descriptions of real-world scenarios to help you learn to identify and understand your responses to various types of psychological trauma.

What is trauma? I'm glad you asked.

It's that feeling that makes your brain and soul feel like they were just hit by an eighteen-wheeler.

And put in a blender.

And then tossed off a ten-story building.

It's the recurrent bad dream that seems to linger in your subconscious.

It's the overwhelming, debilitating stress that overrides our ability to cope, manage, or think clearly.

That is trauma.

Welcome to an elite club— humanity.

Sound like anything you or anyone you know experienced at some point throughout life? Well, if you have never felt like this, consider yourself part of a rare, superhuman minority. On the other hand, if you have felt like this at any point in your life, welcome to an elite club: humanity.

As a psychologist, I am trained to treat trauma as the serious mental health concern that it is. As a human being, prior to my education, I always associated "trauma" with combat veterans and people who experienced heinous incidents like a violent sexual assault, home invasion, or natural disasters.

Through conducting psychotherapy with clients, I've had the opportunity to listen to and protect people's innermost thoughts, struggles, and emotions. I've gained their trust while they've shared with me the behaviors and feelings that have caused them pain, shame, guilt, and feelings of worthlessness. And though it has been challenging for me, at times, to hold their emotions and support them in their quest to develop genuine self-acceptance, inner resolve, and tenacity, I am always ready for a challenge. After all, it's often said that psychologists get into the mental health field to heal their own trauma. I know I did.

Most people have experienced different types of trauma with varying levels of intensity, and we've all been impacted in every major category, including:

- Acute;
- Chronic; and
- Complex.

Acute trauma is known as the "Big T." It describes single events that are painfully unforgettable moments, such as war, sexual abuse, violent attacks, a major car accident or plane crash, robbery, and murder. The "Big T" undercuts the feelings of control and power that are so important to succeeding in life.

Chronic and complex traumas often occur together and come from persistent, more frequent traumatic moments. They are normally labels attached to abuse stemming from those with whom people have long-term connections:

- Child abuse;
- Bad romantic relationships;
- Domestic abuse;
- Abandonment by parents;
- Bullying by siblings; and
- Longtime involvement in a cult.

Trauma can also come from abusive behavior, life conditions, and stress. Additionally, if someone regularly watches bad things happen to other people, that creates trauma.

I'll use myself as an example for this one—time to rip off the Band-Aid. I grew up in a household with a strange dichotomy. My parents were both overprotective *and* negligent. There was no in-between. Let me explain. My parents struggled with drug and alcohol addiction, at different times, throughout their lives. Their drug and alcohol addiction was a symptom of their own childhood trauma. They wanted to break the cycle of abuse and addiction that they had observed in their childhood with their own parents. Having a child was a time of both excitement and fear for them. They wanted to do better than their parents, and in many ways, they did.

The dichotomy was confusing. On one end of the spectrum, they could be negligent of me, and on the other end of the spectrum, they could be overprotective. When my parents were doing well—and by doing well I mean when they were not drinking or using drugs—they were consistent, thoughtful, and engaged parents. My mom could even be described as overprotective. Any time I wanted to go outside and play with my friends, she had to know who I was hanging out with, where I was going, and she made sure that I checked in every hour. I distinctly remember her standing at the top of my street and whistling for me. No matter where I was in the neighborhood, I could hear her whistle. That was my cue to get my butt home.

Now that I am a parent myself, I can appreciate how my parents used the mistakes they made in their lives as teaching moments for me. They were very good at talking *with* me (not *at* me) about topics that make most parents cringe, such as avoiding drugs and alcohol, and how raging hormones can lead to sex and all the responsibilities that go with it. My dad shared stories about the mistakes he made in his own life to help guide me down a better, smarter path. My mom was a nervous Nellie; her anxiety and concern for me were evident. When I was a toddler, I experienced frequent fainting spells that left my parents, especially my mother, in a constant state of worry for me. My mom turned to medical books for answers because so many specialists could not figure out what was wrong with me. Her persistence with the providers at St. Christopher's Hospital for Children in Philadelphia finally paid off. A decade and a half-dozen inaccurate diagnoses later, I was finally diagnosed with *vasovagal syncope*, a condition that is often triggered by heat, dehydration, the sight of blood, and high levels of stress (no surprise there!).

My parents tried their best to raise me in an environment that was better than those from which they came, homes where their parents would drink excessively and then become violent with each other. However, for my father, the violence trickled down to him and his siblings. I remember my dad talking in a humorous manner about how his mother had the unique skill of throwing shoes, wooden spoons, coffee cups, and glasses around corners, hitting them on various body parts from their heads to their stomachs to teach his brothers and sisters a lesson. The point being, violence had been commonplace at home, and my parents didn't want to repeat the same pattern. Unfortunately, wishful thinking doesn't always translate into action.

Negligence is the other side of the dichotomous relationship I experienced with my parents. While binge drinking was my mother's escape from anxiety, it was a reoccurring night terror for me. When my mother drank, I would experience an array of emotions that went from fear to anger to disgust. Truth be told, I never really gave my own feelings related to my mother's drinking and father's violent behavior much thought, if any. My focus was on trying to keep the peace by stopping my parents from killing each other—yes, literally.

Every few weeks, my mom would sneak to the liquor store and buy a pint of Canadian Windsor that she would day-drink. When she drank, I had a constant feeling in the pit in my stomach. Because with every passing hour, my father was closer to coming home. And when he came home and saw my mother drunk, war began.

Outside her drinking benders, my mother was an obedient and hardworking wife. I grew up in the 1980s in Philadelphia, born to an Italian American mother and a Scotch-Irish American father, so using the word *obedient* to describe my mother's role in their marriage is sadly accurate. She was an excellent hairstylist who loved her work. The height of my mom's career was in the 1970s and 1980s; perms, dye jobs, and wash and sets were how she earned her living. The majority of her clients were mature Jewish women from the northeast section of Philadelphia. They loved my mom and how beautiful she made them feel. I can vividly remember their sky-high, teased towers of hair built with equal parts of her talents and AquaNet hair spray. She was a talented hairstylist and tried to be a good mom. But her mental health concerns and drinking consistently got in the way. Her inconsistency was consistent.

When she drank, she had two different personalities: part Beyoncé and part Sasha Fierce. And when she drank, believe me, she was fierce. And fiery. And downright belligerent. Drinking gave her the guts to express how she felt to my father, things she could and would never say while sober. The saying "Some things are better left not said" defined my mom's filter—make that lack of one—when drinking.

When my father returned from work, the fighting would start. At first it would be verbal arguments. They fought about my father's past infidelities, about finances, family—nothing was off limits. I remember sitting on the floor between them while my father screamed at my mother from his chair and my mother lay on the couch yelling back. My head was on a swivel as it went back and forth, watching for one of them to change their posture or get up so I could separate them. Once again, wishful thinking doesn't always translate into action. My father was 6'2" and 300 pounds while my mother weighed in at 110 pounds, 5'5". Once he got up from the chair, I knew it was over. He would punch my mother in the face like she was a man of his size.

Witnessing this kind of violence again and again was traumatizing. Even though my parents never put their hands on me, I witnessed my father do it to my mother. Every time it ended, we were all left crying. I cried because of the fear my father evoked in me, and my mother cried because of the physical and emotional pain he inflicted on her. And my father cried because of the hurt he caused me and my mother. He hated himself because, just like his parents, he so often turned to violence and hurt the people he loved most.

In those moments, I felt alone, scared, and invisible. There was so much rage in my father that he didn't hear me screaming at the top of my lungs for him to stop hitting my mom. And my mom was so drunk that she forgot all about me. The abuse I witnessed left me feeling neglected and alone.

There is another kind of trauma called historical, collective, or intergenerational trauma, which is a shared trauma caused to a generation by an event. Jewish survivors of the Holocaust during World War II, for instance, experienced this type of trauma. After the concentration camps were liberated, the nightmare wasn't over. The survivors had to learn how to live because for so long they had merely been surviving. When freed, their days and nights were filled with reminders of their imprisonment, sleep disturbances, and night terrors.

> Our brains' thoughts and behaviors change when we experience significant trauma.

Without boring you with arcane elements of neuroscience, our brains' thoughts and behaviors change when we experience significant trauma. Even more intriguing is evidence that suggests that trauma experienced by Holocaust survivors could have been passed on to future generations.

Rachel Yehuda, PhD, a world-renowned expert in researching post-traumatic stress disorder (PTSD), has helped us understand the neuroscience of trauma and stress. Dr. Yehuda conducted a study[1] on thirty-two Jewish men and women who had been imprisoned in a Nazi concentration camp, observed or survived heinous torture, or went into hiding during World War II. She analyzed the genes of their children and found that they had an increased likelihood of developing a stress disorder in comparison to the children of Jewish families who escaped Europe during World War II.

Vicarious trauma is also known as secondary trauma. Much like secondhand smoke, this trauma is created by someone hearing about traumatic events from others and becoming traumatized or seeing someone be traumatized and becoming profoundly impacted by it.

Finally, there is "Little T" trauma. This could be labeled *life-change trauma*. With life-change trauma, we experience a major life disruption, such as the loss of a loved one or a job, buying a new home, divorce or breakup, career change, illness, losing a business, transition from high school to college, the process of "coming out," and parenting.

Let's pause for a moment to talk about that last one. Can you think of a career that requires absolutely zero training, that is accompanied by zero vacation days and zero salary? I can. It's called parenting. Many of us do it, but 99.99 percent of us begin the task with no previous training. Sure, some of us have read *What to Expect When You're Expecting, Raising Good Humans,* and *How to Stop Losing Your Sh*t with Your Kids,* which can all be helpful. But the truth is parenting can be traumatic—period. And guess what? It's okay.

When I think about the parenting advice I received, I have a flashback to the "advice cards" that family members and friends filled out for me at my baby shower. They wrote things like "Remember to give your baby tummy time and sleep when the baby sleeps," which is great advice. However, the advice didn't extend through the baby's life span. My son is in middle school now, and I could surely use some "advice cards" to help me get through this phase of his life without ending up as the star character on a true-crime television show. No one really explains how our adorable, chubby-cheeked babies eventually morph into some sort of aliens during their prepubescent and teenage years, and wreak havoc by creating high levels of stress for their caregivers.

Have you ever heard the saying "bigger kids, bigger problems"? When our kids are little we worry about them falling at the playground and eating enough nutritious foods so that they grow and meet their developmental milestones. As our kids get older we also worry about them banging their heads but not at the playground. We worry about teenage kids driving without a seat belt, and the "crowd" they are hanging with. When our kids experience their first heartbreak, it feels like our hearts are broken too. When they are stressed out about getting accepted into their first-choice university, making the travel baseball team, or landing their first "real" job, we are feeling stressed right alongside them. But, most of all, we worry about our children's health and happiness because we know how cruel this world can be. If you have created an environment where your kids feel comfortable talking with you about their worries and struggles, congratulations—you've done an awesome job! But—here's the but—this means that worry has become your default state of existence.

Being a parent can be overwhelming, stressful, anger provoking, and heartbreaking. Parenting is all these things because we do love our kids and we want what's best for them, even though it sometimes takes every last drop of our willpower to not permanently join the witness protection program. But that is not an option. As parents, it's our job to help our kids navigate the world. No matter how old your kids may be, you will always be their parent.

All the traumas mentioned, from Big T to Little T and everything in between, add up and may lead to some of us having significant, lifelong consequences. The difference between the two is resilience, the ability to endure the tough times—and hopefully learn from the challenges.

Why such a range of impacts?

Because we're different in what troubles us and in recognizing or acknowledging what's happening to us. Whether it's a case of not being in touch with our feelings and emotions, listening to and believing the internal, negative self-talk that plays on repeat in our heads, or not knowing how to identify trauma and the mental health responses related to it, trauma has an effect, and we all process it differently.

Surviving traumatic events, like the loss of a partner or recovering from addiction, starts with ensuring that basic human needs (food, shelter, and safety) are met. You can't heal if you don't have the necessities of life.

Here's a good example. My friend Yvonne is a mother of two. Over the past year, Yvonne has been going through a hostile divorce. Her former partner, Michelle, cleaned out their savings account and took off with the family vehicle. Michelle was the primary breadwinner and has stopped supporting Yvonne and their two young children in every sense of the word. Now Yvonne finds herself cleaning houses sixty hours a week to support her children. Maintaining a roof over their heads and feeding and clothing them has left Yvonne no time or opportunity to address the trauma of the breakup because she has been dumped into a new wave of stress. Make sense? Moving from one major trauma to a different type of trauma allows for no healing.

Remember, any of these types of traumas may be deflected when they happen, but the effects tend to boomerang, circling back to smack you in the head so much later that you struggle to uncover a causal relationship between the trauma and that delayed effect. But that effect, however long it may take to surface, is aftershock.

How Our Unmet Needs Can Cause Aftershock

It is nearly impossible to address mental health problems when the basics of life are threatened. In fact, as you will recall, part of what defines post-traumatic stress disorder is the need to bury our emotions lest they overwhelm our ability to address life-threatening situations; later, those emotions may surface in ways that damage our mental health. You also know that this same "bury our emotions" response can lead to a subclinical form of post-traumatic stress response that I call aftershock.

The most basic levels of needs are physiological needs or the must-haves, which were famously outlined years ago by American psychologist Abraham Maslow; I mean, this wouldn't be a psychology book without a mention of Maslow's Hierarchy of Needs.

Maslow was a brilliant psychologist who developed his Hierarchy of Needs in 1943. The hierarchy is a chart of human needs that people must achieve to realize their full potential and appreciation for life, ranging from the most basic requirements for survival to self-actualization—a fancy way of defining the motivations that help us realize our full potential. But here's the kicker: according to Dr. Maslow, each need builds upon the other, starting with our most basic or must-have needs like food, water, and shelter, all the way up to our higher-level needs, like building mutual respect with others, self-esteem, morality, and creativity.[2]

When our must-have needs are threatened, it's difficult to focus on anything else.

You're probably familiar with the expression "living from paycheck to paycheck"? That was exactly how we lived when I was a child. My father was a self-employed brick mason, and my mother, as you know, was a hairstylist. You might assume that they would have no problem making ends meet, but they struggled financially. Winters were the worst for my father's business as freezing temperatures don't lend themselves to cement mixing and bricklaying. Then again, even when the weather cooperated, balancing a checkbook wasn't one of my father's strong suits either.

I remember times when my parents would count loose change to buy eggs and bread. There were also times when they would ask to "borrow" birthday money I had received from my grandmother to pay the water or gas bill. Paying rent for our modest apartment was also a challenge. My parents would often fall behind and find themselves asking family members to help them avoid eviction. The dichotomy in my house was evident, even when it came to finances; there was no in-between. We either ate like royalty or survived on ramen noodles. And I'm not talking about the fancy ramen with the boiled eggs, steak, and diced green onions that I keep seeing on TikTok. I'm talking about the 10 cents a pack, beef-flavored ramen that you find on the bottom shelf of the soup aisle at the grocery store. You can say that sometimes our must-haves were more like have-nots.

As an adult, I have thought about how struggling to meet our basic needs impacted my parents (let's leave how it impacted me out of this for now). Did it stunt their ability to work on higher-level needs like love, belonging, and self-esteem? Was it traumatic to be in a constant state of stress, trying to ensure that our basic needs were met? The short answer is yes.

When must-have needs like food, shelter, and safety are consistently threatened, our minds don't have the luxury of fulfilling other needs, according to our dear Dr. Maslow. For example, because my parents consistently struggled to simply survive and make ends meet, there was little energy expended on esteem needs, such as achieving a sense of accomplishment and positive self-worth, and self-actualizing needs, such as personal growth.

So how did my parents cope with the stress of trying to have their must-have needs met? They argued. My mother tried to escape, if even for a short time, by forming an unhealthy relationship with alcohol. My father became violent. And they argued some more. When our needs aren't met, we may turn to unhealthy ways of coping. Now, do I think that the deficit in having their needs met was the cause of all their problems? No. But I do think that it contributed to the high stress levels in our home.

Let's stick with my parents as we climb our way to the middle of Maslow's Hierarchy of Needs. Above our physiological/security needs, which we have already referred to as the must-have needs (food, water, shelter, and safety), are our social needs, which include belonging, love, and family/friends. We've established that my parents had a hard time meeting their basic needs, which made it challenging to work their way up Maslow's pyramid. Though I appreciate Dr. Maslow's theory, I think that it is important to note that people can move up and down Maslow's Hierarchy of Needs throughout their lives.

My parents vacillated between trying to meet their basic needs and their need for love and belonging. I think they sometimes even attempted to fulfill both sets of needs simultaneously. When we had a little money—when the bills were paid, the refrigerator was packed, and the rent was up-to-date—the stress related to our must-haves decreased. My parents could take a much-needed sigh of relief. But when the feeling of relief from the burden of financial stress was lifted, it was quickly replaced with arguments about their marriage. Who cheated when and with whom?

Neither of them genuinely felt loved by the other; their love came with many conditions and contingencies because their relationship wasn't a trusting one. They no longer trusted each other with their feelings. And that void was filled with alcohol, Percocet, and, ironically enough, infidelity.

> The human species requires the need to feel understood and connected to others.

After all, the human species requires the need to feel understood and connected to others. As much as our fellow humans possess the innate gift of effortlessly making us cry, we relentlessly get back up, dry our tears, and continue our quest to feel loved and accepted.

As we continue our climb up Dr. Maslow's pyramid, our needs become more sophisticated. Esteem needs include self-confidence, achievement, self-worth, and respect for and by others. And finally, at the very top of the pyramid, we have self-actualization needs, which is a fancy way of explaining the ability to meet our full potential. When I think of esteem and self-actualization needs, I think of Greg, my husband.

Let me give you a little context and take a moment to introduce you all to my husband—or, as I like to call him, "Moose," because he loves to eat! Aside from his insatiable appetite and handsome looks, Greg comes from an athletically gifted family. He has two older brothers who played competitive soccer and kicked for Division II football teams in college.

Greg was a skilled soccer and basketball player, and he played for the Sonny Hill Community Basketball League in Philadelphia. Mr. Hill credits Greg and his brothers for desegregating his league, as they were the first, and for some time the only, white kids who played for Mr. Hill. Greg even played AAU hoops with Kobe Bryant for Mr. Sam Rines' James Fox Basketball League. He played in high school and went on to play Division II basketball at East Stroudsburg University before transferring to Millersville University and ultimately ending his college career at Keane University. After graduating, he played pro ball for the Washington Generals (one of the teams that plays against the Harlem Globetrotters), playing ninety-six games in one hundred days. Greg ate, slept, and breathed basketball. It was and may arguably still be his first love (don't worry, I've accepted it).

He loved the game and put so much pressure on himself to be the best. If practice ended at 6 PM, Greg stayed at the gym until 8 PM, practicing his shot. He went to the gym daily to weight train and woke up early every morning to run before class. He spent so much time on basketball that it consumed him.

When I talk with Greg about that time in his life, he explains that he thought he was "letting people down" by not realizing his full potential at the college level. A lack of effort and dedication to honing his skills could not be blamed for his lack of self-confidence; he lived at the gym! So what was it?

Several things were going on. The coaches who recruited him to play found opportunities elsewhere, leaving Greg with a new coach who saw him as the "old coach's" recruit. He was fearful of the unknown with his new coach. Would his role on the team change? Would the new coach value him like his previous coach? Would he get enough playing time? Would the new coach like him or try to get rid of him? Then, unfortunately for Greg, he suffered a right ankle injury, torn abdominal muscle, and inguinal hernia while trying to navigate the already difficult season. The injuries instilled further doubt in Greg as to whether his feet would hit the court.

Greg's dedication and commitment to basketball didn't fade. He rehabbed his ankle and abdomen and got back to practicing with his team as quickly as he could. He even continued to practice on his own, waking up at 5:00 AM, running through drills, and relentlessly trying to perfect his game. However, the hours of practice and conditioning failed to make Greg feel any better. He wasn't getting playing time, despite his efforts. Perhaps he was too ambitious to expect to play right after his injury? After all, he was eligible to play for several more years, so if this wasn't the year for him to get ample playing time, the following year could be different.

But the pressure Greg put on himself did not allow him to look at his situation through that lens. He felt like he was failing and, in turn, failing everyone around him. Greg's esteem needs were not being met, according to our buddy Dr. Maslow. He was struggling with the side effects or repercussions of multiple Little T traumas, for example, suffering multiple physical injuries as a dedicated college athlete, transferring to three different schools to increase his chances for more playing time, and maintaining good grades. He felt like he was failing to accomplish his main goal at that time, which was to be a successful college basketball player, and his feelings of failure took a significant toll on his self-esteem. His struggle to fulfill his esteem needs prevented him from realizing his full potential or self-actualizing needs.

So what did this struggle look like for Greg—how did it impact him? The pressure he placed on himself became insurmountable. And his internal monologue (or little dictator, as I like to call it) morphed into a total asshole that put him down and pulverized any semblance of self-worth he had left. Public enemy number one for most of us is (drumroll please) ourselves.

All that negative self-talk from his little dictator started to affect Greg; he started believing that he wasn't good enough and that he was failing everyone he loved. He ended up getting severely depressed, but the people around Greg didn't have an inkling about what was going on inside his head. They didn't know how he felt because everything appeared copacetic to the outside world.

While struggling with depression, he continued to attend classes, work out, eat well, and earn a 3.5 GPA. You would never have known the internal struggle he was having because the typical or apparent signs/symptoms of depression were not evident with Greg. What people didn't know or see was that his sleep schedule was atypical. He found himself sleeping at off hours and isolating himself from his teammates and peers at school. He was living with feelings of guilt and had difficulty concentrating.

I remember him telling me that it took him nearly three hours to finish his history midterm because he had such a challenging time concentrating. He read each question multiple times because he was unable to comprehend what was being asked and had trouble deciding which multiple-choice answers to select. This may not seem like a big deal, but the inability to concentrate and focus because of the noise produced by your own negative self-talk is frightening.

After his midterm, he drove home from college and asked his parents for help. Blindsided by this revelation, they got Greg the mental health help he needed.

More than two decades later, I look at Greg with genuine admiration. I admire the strength he exhibited in asking for help. I admire how he has dedicated himself to his mental health the same way he dedicated himself to basketball. His commitment to his mental health has afforded him the opportunity to be the best version of himself, which has been inspiring to witness.

Today, he is a supportive, loving, and, might I say, hilarious husband and father. He also has the best job in the world. He gets to wake up every day, throw on basketball shorts and sneakers, and teach health and physical education to middle schoolers. I know that some of you reading this are probably cringing and thinking, *Eww, middle school?* Yet, despite the pervasive smell of prepubescent body odor mixed with raging hormones, Greg loves teaching them. His life experience (or trauma) has given him grace and the ability to share it with the kids he teaches during a time in their lives when they are all trying to find their way.

Tying It All Together

As Dr. Maslow explained to us, human needs encompass a broad spectrum ranging from the must-haves to finding our purpose and realizing our potential. Greg was struggling to realize his own purpose and meet his full potential in the same way that my parents struggled to find safety and belongingness. In other words, everyone experiences high levels of stress at different periods in life, and the interpretation of that stress varies from person to person.

The saying "first-world problems" is one that I sometimes use when I find myself commiserating over something with my best friend, Sue, who you'll get to learn more about a little later. Recently, we were having a conversation about some of the characters at Sue's job who have an uncanny way of throwing more work at Sue while simultaneously complaining about how stressed out they are at the job. Sound familiar to anyone?

In the thick of our conversation, I could tell that Sue was stressed out. She had been working painfully long hours in an effort to remedy the issues at her workplace and felt as though she was getting nowhere; kind of like trying to sprint through quicksand. I listened to her and tried to be supportive, mostly by using inappropriate and dark humor.

Toward the end of our conversation, she said, "I should shut up. These are all first-world problems!" However, our dear friend Dr. Maslow would put it slightly differently: "Sue, you are feeling stressed because you are having a difficult time getting your high-level needs met."

At first, we chuckled about this, but then I thought about it a little bit more. Why should Sue or any of us dismiss or minimize our stress because we think it pales in comparison to people who have "real problems"? I get it: Sue didn't want to come off as a whiner or complainer. She wanted reassurance by reminding herself that there are people out there who struggle to have their must-have needs met. This is a valid point. And it is understandable for us to compare ourselves to people who are less fortunate than we are in some distorted attempt to remind us to be grateful for what we have. But let's be real for a minute: That doesn't work in the long run. It might work for us temporarily, after we say it out loud, but the truth is that we don't live other people's lives; we live our own lives. What causes me stress in my life may not be even a blip on someone else's stress-o-meter. But that doesn't make it irrelevant.

Trauma is an inescapable part of the human experience that we will all encounter at some point.

After all, trauma is defined as a deeply distressing or disturbing experience. And what is deeply distressing and disturbing for one person may not be the same for another. Trauma should not be reserved for the *Diagnostic and Statistical Manual for Psychiatric Disorders* (DSM). Just because someone experiences trauma and has a psychological response to it does not warrant a diagnosis of a mental illness or disorder. Trauma is an inescapable part of the human experience that we will all encounter at some point.

Similarly, just because you don't suffer from PTSD does not mean that the trauma you've experienced has had no lasting ill effects on your mental health. Even if you "only" suffer from aftershock as the result of stressful events that were not quite stressful enough to cause PTSD, it can make your life far more painful and difficult than it should be. My advice is to buckle up, buttercups, because it is going to be a crazy ride!

SO LET'S REVIEW:

Dr. Maslow's Hierarchy of Needs incorporates basic needs like food, safety, and rest; psychological needs like close relationships and a sense of accomplishment; and self-fulfillment needs like reaching your full potential.

People can move up and down Maslow's Hierarchy of Needs throughout their lives.

Your needs are not to be compared with others' needs. It makes no difference if you are struggling with a must-have need or a "psychological" need. If it causes you stress, it is relevant.

Experiencing persistent and/or high levels of stress is traumatic. But it does not mean that you have post-traumatic stress disorder.

Being human equates to experiencing traumatic events throughout our lives and that's okay. Because resilience is born out of trauma.

There are many different types of trauma, from complex trauma to vicarious trauma.

Within every flavor of trauma, there are varying levels of severity.

Resilience speaks to a person's ability to cope with trauma.

Fulfilling our basic needs is obviously necessary for survival.

Meeting your basic needs, controlling what you can control, and being kind to yourself can help you survive.

CHAPTER TWO

How Trauma Shapes Who We Are

TRAUMA IS NOT JUST SIMPLY a psychological disorder. It is a part of the human condition—shitty but unavoidable—and classifying an individual's response to trauma as a mental disorder may be inaccurate. Trauma responses are due to psychological injury, not psychopathology. The severity of traumatic events varies, as do an individual's responses to them.

We might often hear the phrase "They were traumatized." When we dig a little deeper, we learn that this phrase has been applied to an array of incidents, from a nasty divorce to the loss of parent/caregiver. Granted, we tend to freely throw this term around for minor hiccups in life as much as we do for shockingly distressful events. The point being is that a person's response to what they *perceive* as trauma varies based on many factors, such as their character, personality traits, how they grew up in regard to relationships with caregivers, environment, financial means, and the trauma itself. Trauma and our responses to it are unique.

Personality Traits

Personality theory has been researched and analyzed for decades. I'm sure you have heard of Sigmund Freud, known as the father of modern psychology. For those of us who have studied Freud, we also credit him with making recreational use of cocaine popular in the late 1800s.[3] (What kind of scientist would he be if he didn't test his product, right?) He penned a paper titled "Uber Coca" in which he describes cocaine's exhilarating euphoric effect, suppression of fatigue and hunger, and let's not forget, its ability to stave off depression. Sounds like a dream—no pun intended. But here's the catch: Our buddy Freud missed the boat on cocaine's addictive properties, despite his own dependence. This oversight might impart some doubt regarding Dr. Freud's credibility as one of the greatest psychological minds of our time, but look at it this way: Most brilliant people are a little nuts. Or a lot. At any rate, I like to include this ironic detail about Freud to show that even highly accomplished people don't always have it together.

Dr. Freud was an Austrian neurologist whose curiosity about the human psyche led to the development of psychoanalysis, which is a fancy way of stating that humans have thoughts, feelings, memories, and desires that we repress or shut off. Dr. Freud developed psychoanalysis to help bring those repressed feelings to light by having patients talk freely and openly with a focus on early childhood experiences. So you can thank Freud for psychologists' compulsion to dig into your childhood. Believe it or not, there is a strategy behind why we ask about the relationships and experiences you had with early caregivers. It helps us understand your personality and, in turn, your behaviors.

Relationships

Early relationships shape our personalities. Whether we want to accept it or not, as parents we are charged with the responsibility of guiding, teaching, and instilling values and beliefs in our children. Some psychological theories describe a new life or young child's personality as a tabula rasa, which is Latin for "blank slate." In other words, children learn how to view the world, themselves, and others from their parents.

The role of a parent or caregiver isn't something we get to train for; there is no parenting academy or school to attend before becoming a parent. Believe me, if such a school existed, I would be first in line with my tuition check in hand.

As much as we try to protect our kids and do our best parenting, at times we fall flat on our faces. Yup—we will undoubtedly do or say things that upset our kids. For most of us, it's not intentional; it's inadvertent. Will we also nurture, protect, and help our children develop into productive adults? Yes!

But let's be real. Parenting is not 9 to 5; it is 24/7. We will have bad days, times when our parenting may be questionable.

And that's okay. According to another psychoanalyst, Dr. Donald Winnicott, who was also a pediatrician, "good enough parenting" means that you're meeting your child's needs just 30 percent of the time.[4] He believes that's sufficient for children to become happy and well-attached. Hopefully, this gives all you parents out there a big sigh of relief. "Perfect parenting" can be counterproductive because it means children are never given the opportunity to face adversity. So all of you high achievers out there can take a back seat while the rest of us enjoy this guilt-free victory lap of subpar parenting.

Resilience

Making mistakes due to our emotions, losing one's cool, and feeling significantly overwhelmed or stressed out are normal emotions that we can't always tuck away in some hidden internal compartment. Whether it is that annoying neighbor knocking on your door with their list of grievances, your partner, an egomaniacal boss, kids (of all ages), or a mentally draining sibling, it can be difficult to manage our own emotions and our responses to how others are interacting with us.

> Losing one's cool or feeling overwhelmed are normal emotions that we can't always tuck away . . .

In plain English, when we are stressed, we say and do things that cause others psychic pain. It comes down to relationships, how we interact with others, and how others interact with us that help to build and shape how we view ourselves and our world. We are all going to treat someone in our lives poorly, even though we may not intentionally set out to hurt them. It is inevitable, kind of like breaking your New Year's resolution after just three weeks. And guess what? It's okay. No, seriously, it's okay because many of the fumbles we make as parents, partners, daughters, sons, siblings, and friends teach us *resilience*. The American Psychological Association (APA)[5] defines resilience as the process and outcome of successfully adapting to difficult or challenging life experiences, especially through mental, emotional, and behavioral flexibility and adjustment to external and internal demands.

You may have heard the Japanese proverb "Fall down seven times, get up eight," or the wise words of Roy T. Bennet, famous author and Zimbabwean politician: "It doesn't matter how many times you fall down, it's how many times you get up." These both explain resilience. Here's the thing about resilience: She makes you work very hard to be her friend. Not everyone is worthy of her friendship, even though all of us have fallen more times than we would like to admit.

JERRY'S STORY

Folks who know me well also know that I have always looked up to my dad, Jerry Utter. Not so much in the sense that I wanted to be like him, but more in the spirit of wanting to be loved and accepted by him. I wanted to make him proud of me. Don't worry, we will dig into my "daddy issues" shortly.

My dad had a very charismatic personality that was complemented by a combination of Richard Pryor's and George Carlin's senses of humor. He was blessed with the innate ability to captivate people's attention. He just had a way of talking that made people want to listen. He also had a mean set of singing pipes. Anyway, from the time I was a young child, the old man would talk with me about life and topics that most parents avoid like the plague. I had VIP status and a front-row seat into learning about how my father's colorful life, fueled by drugs, sex, and rock 'n' roll, led to poor decisions and negative consequences that he paid the price for throughout his life.

One of eight children, Jerry was raised during the 1950s and 1960s in what was once a working-class area of Philadelphia famously known as Kensington. Today, Kensington is renowned for its open-air drug market, which predominantly offers illicitly manufactured fentanyl. Jerry's father, Bob, was a WWII Navy veteran, factory worker, and political ward leader in his district. His mother, Marg, tended bar but spent much of her time raising a gaggle of kids. Bob and Marg met after WWII when Marg was tending bar at a local corner bar. At that time, Marg was a newly divorced mother of three, one boy and two girls. Her ex-husband was verbally and emotionally abusive, and he hit Marg almost as hard as he hit the bottle.

When she met Bob, there was an immediate attraction. The two began to date and shortly thereafter bought a house on Mascher Street. At the time, Marg's three children from her previous marriage were living in a group home because she was unable to care for them. When she and Bob got together, she managed to regain custody of her children. Over the next few years, Marg gave birth to five more children: Nancy, Robert Jr., Jerome (Jerry), and twins Denise and Roxanne. Raising eight children in a small home on a modest income was a strain. In turn, Bob drank more while Marg began to take her frustration out on the kids.

The five younger children, including my father, received the brunt of Marg's wrath—she's the one I mentioned who had the skill of throwing shoes, glasses, coffee mugs, and basically anything she could get her hands on, around a corner. NFL teams could have used her as a quarterback!

Every night Marg peeled at least ten pounds of potatoes as they were a cheap and filling staple side dish in the Utter household. One night, while peeling every inch of skin off the potatoes with a paring knife, Bobby, Jerry's brother, talked back to Marg. Now, if you know anything about growing up in the sixties, you know that talking back to your parents, or any adult, for that matter, was not tolerated. In true Marg fashion, she threatened to smack Bobby in the mouth if he didn't lay off the back talk, to which Bobby replied with snark. Marg then psyched Bobby out and acted as if she were going to throw the paring knife at him. Naturally, he jumped, thinking that he dodged the knife, but Bobby didn't realize that Marg was a step ahead of him. As Bobby's feet hit the floor, thinking that he beat Marg at her own game, she threw the knife, hitting Bobby in his upper left thigh!

Watching his brother fall to the floor in pain, my father ran over to help him. Marg responded by throwing my father in the

basement with no lights. My father was afraid of the dark, and
Marg was well aware of this fear. Meanwhile, Bobby removed the
paring knife from his leg and nursed his wound.

Shortly thereafter Jerry and Bobby's father came home from
work. He saw what had happened to Bobby's leg and learned that
my father was locked in the basement. He immediately unlocked
the basement door, got my father out, and checked on Bobby's
wound. After making sure his sons were okay, he and Marg
argued. And once they started to argue, it was only a matter of
time before fists began to fly.

Marg is undeniably the villain in this story. Physical violence
coupled with verbal assaults from Marg were commonplace in my
father's childhood home. Marg was a bully. She would call him
names like "Dumbo" because he had big ears. This was not delivered in a cutesy manner; she called him Dumbo to hurt him.

Bullies are not just school-age peers;
they can be coworkers, employers, and even
your own parents. My father also struggled
academically; he had a hard time reading.
I remember him sharing with me that if it
were not for his ability to draw, he would
not have gotten through middle school.
My father would make handmade holiday
decorations for his classroom, and because
of his artistic talent, his teachers promoted
him to the next grade. He didn't have any support. Rather than
give him the help he needed to succeed, his mother teased him

and called him stupid. In ninth grade, my father dropped out of school. He never received the academic support he needed because his mother, rather than advocating for him, bullied him about his learning differences instead.

The way she treated her children is inexcusable. However, mentioning that she too was the victim of physical and verbal abuse by her parents and former husband might solicit feelings of sympathy, even comfort, because it helps to give us a plausible, humane explanation for the behavior she displayed with her own children. The intent of sharing my father's story is to demonstrate how relationships and interactions with our caregivers can affect our personalities in the long term. Our interactions, especially those that are negative or traumatizing, are the precursors that lay the foundation for how we perceive ourselves, others, and the world. Bad life experiences are part of the secret sauce that builds resilience.

My father had many redeeming qualities. He was charismatic, outgoing, a dapper dresser, and quite comical. He also possessed other qualities that were correlated to the way his sense of self was nurtured (or more like *not* nurtured) by his caregivers, peers, and those closest to him. For example, because he was teased by his mother and his peers about his physical appearance (remember they called him Dumbo), he felt self-conscious about his looks. My dad was ridiculed at home and school for his learning differences; reading was challenging. So as a young child, the manner in which he viewed himself was less than, not good or bad. Dr. Freud would be tempted to posit that my dad struggled with introjection, an ego defense mechanism that occurs when an individual internalizes or believes the opinions or viewpoint of other people.[6] This set the stage for how he viewed the world: as a place where he could not trust or show vulnerability.

Humor and taking pride in his physical appearance were defense mechanisms used by my father and demonstrations of his resilience. As I analyze my father's response to the traumas he has experienced, I can't help but think of our friend Dr. Freud as he hypothesized that the expression of humor helps to transform the damaging psychological effect of a threatening situation into a pleasurable experience.[7] A perfect example of how he used humor was when he first told me the story about Marg slinging a paring knife at his brother. We were practically in tears laughing because he told the story the same way stand-up comedians deliver bits to an audience. Regarding his looks, puberty worked its magic, and he ended up going from a scrunty, big-eared kid to a 6'2" swarthy bass baritone. His drive to look his best all the time was correlated with his subconscious need to cancel out his childhood experiences that made him feel like the ugly duckling. Taking pride in his physical appearance and his use of pithy humor are demonstrations of resilience.

However, my father also adopted less-than-optimal coping strategies. Alcohol and drug abuse were rampant in his household, though if you asked him, he would downplay it. His father, Bob, was a hardworking man. He provided for his family; however, his Achilles heel was drinking a few whiskeys on ice every evening after work. It seemed harmless, but with the alcohol came domestic violence. His parents got physical with each other in front of my father and his siblings. His mother wasn't much of a drinker, but she indulged in taking diet pills known as black beauties. I'm not talking about over-the-counter diet pills; these were prescribed amphetamines. In the sixties, black beauties weren't believed to be addictive, but they were. So much so that Marg could not function without them. With the verbal and physical abuse that my father both observed and fell victim to, he also began to abuse drugs.

At age eleven, he started huffing paint thinner. At age sixteen, he lost his father to lung cancer due to exposure to asbestos. With his father's death, he went further down the path of drug abuse. There was little guidance in the family home. By the time he was in his late teens, he was shooting heroin. His addiction to heroin influenced criminogenic behaviors, which led to his incarceration. While in jail, he kicked his heroin habit. However, after his release, he moved on to manufacturing and abusing methamphetamines, which eventually led to more time behind bars.

By the time he was in his early thirties, he had stopped abusing drugs. I was around four years old, and it was also around this time that my dad started talking with me about the mistakes he made in life and what he wanted for me. He wanted to prevent me from going down the same path. "Gerawin," he would say, using his nickname for me, "the three most important things in your life are your family, your education, and God."

In some ways, my father succeeded in breaking the cycle of physical and verbal abuse that occurred in his childhood home.

But in other ways, the cycle of trauma continued. The trauma he experienced as a youngster impacted his personality and how he viewed himself, others, and the world. It makes me wonder how my father's life might have been different if he didn't grow up in the household that he did. Did leaning on drugs as a way to cope and escape stunt his ability to pursue his life goals? There were periods in his life when he was simply trying to survive rather than searching for purpose or finding meaning in his life.

The challenging life experiences he had in his early years shaped his personality in positive and negative ways. We tend to focus on how adverse incidents influence unhealthy coping strategies, such as my father's drug abuse. However, we often give less attention to how traumatic experiences help to inspire positive aspects of our personality, such as humor and resilience.

As I got older, my father and I talked about his questionable, though lively, lifestyle, and how it might have been different with a healthier upbringing. At first, I was taken aback by his response. He said, "I wouldn't change a thing. All the shit I went through helped make me who I am."

"You aren't angry or upset with your mom?" I asked. "Resentful about losing your father at such a young age? You never think about how your life might be different if you didn't abuse drugs and alcohol?"

"Of course I have thought about all those things, but the mistakes I have made and the way I was treated by my mother and others close to me taught me what I wanted to do differently with you," he answered.

I admired his ability to accept, forgive, and move past the rotten things he endured, even though some of it was self-induced. But I didn't really understand or appreciate it until I gained more life experience. Not to mention, becoming a shrink has taught me more about trauma and how humans respond to it.

When distressing things happen to us, and they will, we will respond. Some of us respond in negative ways, and some respond in healthy, positive ways. The third option is that we will respond both positively and negatively. My dad adopted that "mixed bag" approach in a big way.

> When distressing things happen to us, and they will, we will respond.

He learned how to use humor and develop a charismatic and outgoing personality to get a reaction from others and his environment that nurtured how he felt about himself. Unfortunately, he also abused drugs and alcohol as a means to cope with and numb the psychological pain associated with his past experiences. His poor self-concept of not feeling good enough damaged him.

However, one of the useful traits that my father learned was resilience. He learned how to navigate the world and find his purpose in life because of his childhood of trauma and distress. My dad learned that it's not about how many times you fall but how many times you get back up.

SO LET'S REVIEW:

A person's character, personality traits, and how they grew up regarding their relationships with caregivers and environment plays a huge role in what they perceive as traumatic.

Trauma and our responses to it are unique. What one person perceives as traumatic may not be a blip on someone else's radar.

Resilience is what helps us adapt to highly stressful life experiences.

Humor and determination can be resilient coping strategies born out of trauma.

Remember the Japanese proverb "Fall down seven times, get up eight."

CHAPTER THREE

Feelings Are
Always to Blame

YES, I WILL BE talking about *feelings*—the other "F" word.

Think of your feelings as your psyche's GPS system. They guide your behavior, mood, and psychological well-being. The tricky thing about feelings is that they sneak up on you. You believe you have gotten past or over a distressing event, then find yourself fighting back tears in the checkout line at Target, painfully aware that you are being watched on security cameras.

Tearfulness, sadness, depression, irritability, anger, and anxiety are only a few of the delayed emotions, or the aftershock, that you might feel weeks, months, or even years after having experienced a traumatic event—or even mundane yet stressful events like a job change. The fact is that when something stressful happens to you, it has an effect on you, although not always immediately. Let me use my mother, Jeanne, to illustrate.

I always joke around with my mother, saying, "I swear you're part cat because you really do have nine lives."

Those who know anything about Jeanne know what I mean. Mom has lived an extremely, um, *colorful* life. She struggled for three decades with opioid addiction and has been in rehab so often that the place should be named after her. She is a fiery, feisty, funny Italian mother. More "F" words! And let me tell you, she smells bullshit a mile away! My mom has the superpower of being able to read someone within five minutes of meeting them, which has helped me avoid some attractive but shady characters in my life (thanks, Mom!). But I would be remiss if I said that our relationship has been all rainbows and kittens; she has often been a handful, and I sometimes feel like the mother rather than the daughter.

Despite the roller coaster of a relationship that we share, I have always had my mother's back. In December 2020, Mom had just completed yet another stint in rehab and didn't want to go back to her apartment to live alone. So my husband and I invited her to live with us and our children, Natalee and Gregory, with the very strict and non-negotiable proviso that she follow two important rules. One: no drugs or alcohol. Two: she had to participate in mental health treatment. We made it clear that there would be no exceptions or second chances! Our children would be under that same roof, and, as protective as I feel about Mom, double that for my kids.

I'm happy to say that, after decades of active addiction, my mom held up her end of the deal. She cooked, helped out with the kids, and had a solid group of sober supports with whom she enjoyed spending time. It looked like life had finally given Jeanne a much-needed respite from the all-consuming chaos that had defined her life for so long.

Life threw her another challenge in June 2022 when her primary care provider ordered a routine mammogram. Begrudgingly, my mother complied but didn't think much about it. About ten days later, she received a call from her doctor. He told her that they had spotted a suspicious mass on her right breast. She waited to share the news with me until Gregory and Natalee went to soccer practice. I immediately went into "self-protective" mode, arguing that we should not anticipate the worst until a biopsy of the mass is taken. I know: easier said than done, right?

Within a week of the biopsy, Mom was scheduled for surgery to remove the mass. We visited the surgeon, Dr. James Moore, who guided us through the process from start to finish. On July 20, she underwent a full right-breast mastectomy. The biopsy results revealed that she had HER2, estrogen-sensitive, stage 2 breast cancer. Keep in mind that only four weeks had passed from diagnosis to surgery. Further analysis of the biopsy revealed the best news possible: She did not need radiation or chemotherapy treatments. She also learned that her reoccurrence score was zero and that her reoccurrence risk at nine years was 3 percent. Talk about a gigantic sigh of relief! Her surgeon even shared with us that throughout his thirty-year career, he had never *seen* a recurrence score of zero! This was the most positive scenario anyone could ask for.

Mom was overwhelmed by this wonderful news. She had been running on adrenaline, operating in "survival mode," and participating in a variety of medical tests and surgery in a mind-numbing effort to extend her life.

And just like that, it was over. She had won her battle. You would assume that she would feel relieved, grateful, happy. And she did. But unfortunately, once the adrenaline subsided, her brain realized that she was no longer in survival mode. In survival mode, we instinctively realize that we'd better keep our heads down and our emotions in check, or we may not survive. But those emotions don't disappear. They simply submerge, waiting for their chance to bubble to the surface and wreak havoc.

> In survival mode, we instinctively realize that we'd better keep our heads down and our emotions in check, or we may not survive.

Imagine a pink balloon, fully inflated, floating in the air. The pink balloon represents you in fight or survival mode. You are fully inflated, armed, and ready to go to war. There isn't time or mental space to worry or be depressed. You put those emotions aside to focus on kicking cancer's ass. Now, picture the pink balloon overinflating, popping, and falling to earth in scattered pieces. That overblown pink balloon represents my mother's emotions after she received her prognosis, but when it burst, the reality of everything that she had been through set in, and the cycle of aftershock emotions began.

I remember Mom feeling fatigued and subdued during the weeks following her excellent cancer prognosis. I also remember her telling me that she felt depressed and couldn't understand why. There were times I observed her quietly crying while washing the dishes or making dinner. As a clinician educated on delayed trauma responses, I could empathize with Mom, but that didn't make it any easier for her to struggle to adjust as her dormant emotions surfaced and rocked her world. Luckily, I was trained to recognize the issue, and time and attention to her mental health helped Mom work through the aftermath of emotions she experienced as a cancer survivor.

I feel like it is important to share with you that, as my mother's main support system, after the danger to her subsided, I too began to feel my emotions spin. Let me explain: Even though my mother was the one who was diagnosed with cancer and had to learn how to navigate the array of pent-up feelings associated with her circumstances, I also felt a burden as her primary support. I want to make clear that you too can feel impacted by a traumatic event that happens to someone you care about; that's *vicarious trauma*.

Like my mother, I was in fight mode, taking her to doctor's appointments, consulting with providers, or offering her a listening ear or an encouraging, "You got this!"

And although it was the least I could do, it left me worried and down once the pressure was off. And guess what? Drum roll, please: it is perfectly okay to feel emotionally beat-up after helping someone through a traumatic time in their life.

But it's also important to understand that, whether you are the victim or the supporter, these are not emotions that you need to manage on your own. Whether you share how you're feeling with a supportive friend or reach out to a trained mental health professional for help, take care of your mental health in the same way you do for others! It is not a little thing to be troubled after you have helped carry a loved one through a fire; the potential for aftershock is real and should not be ignored or dismissed as mere weakness on your part.

> . . . take care of your mental health in the same way you do for others!

And to be transparent, that's exactly what I did. I felt as though I had to remain stoic, upbeat, and positive when I was with Mom, sheltering her from the fear and danger that had exploded into her life. Later, having a safe space in therapy sessions to unload all those emotions finally gave me the opportunity to breathe—to exhale. For a moment, let me hop up on my soapbox: Therapy is not reserved exclusively for folks with severe mental health concerns, such as major depression or schizoaffective disorder. It's for anyone who feels stuck, who wants to improve how they feel about themselves and build up their self-worth, or who desires someone nonjudgmental and engaged to speak with. It's for any of us suffering from aftershock, even if it's not at the level of helping a parent fight cancer! The list goes on, but my point is, therapy is for everyone.

My mom's story is merely an example of the inevitable life events that so many of us will encounter: the death of a parent, miscarriage, illness, parenthood, career changes, death of a spouse or partner, a new career, and marriage. These life events forever change us.

Keep in mind that the way an event affects us—and its severity—varies.

I'll use my mother-in-law, Carol, as an example. After forty years of marriage, my father-in-law, John, suddenly passed away from a blood clot that traveled from his leg to his lungs while playing racquetball. He died instantly.

The terrifying call I received from Greg that his father was found unresponsive at the gym and was being rushed by ambulance to the local hospital is one I will never forget. I met Greg at the hospital, and a short time later we all went back to his family home. His mother, two brothers, relatives, and family friends visited to give their condolences. Throughout the days leading up to John's services, my younger sister, Dominique, and I spent as much time as we could with Greg and his family.

I distinctly remember Carol having to call John's father to tell him the news. Before making the call, she said to her sister, "I can't believe I have to call Jack and tell him that John died." That must have been one of the hardest things she ever had to do. A parent should never have to learn that their child died. She gracefully delivered the worst news imaginable to her father-in-law and grieved with her sons, but I could see that she didn't want them to see just how much pain *she* was in over her husband's death. Even during such a tragic time, she protected her sons from having to worry about her.

At the funeral, there were over a thousand people in attendance at the church. The pews were completely packed, and people lined the perimeter of the church to pay their respects to the family. Carol delivered the eulogy with such strength and love that every person in attendance looked at her with complete admiration; I know I did. The outpouring of support that Carol received at John's funeral speaks to the kind of person he was—genuine, kind, funny, supportive, down-to-earth. Proof that Carol and John made one great pair.

Not only did my mother-in-law handle the days following John's death with grace, but nearly two decades after his passing, she continues to be an independent, hardworking woman who puts her family first, especially her six grandchildren. I'm sure there are times when she cries in private and still experiences the pain of losing her husband and high school sweetheart. Grief does not have an expiration date. Like my mother-in-law, we learn how to live even though life is not the same without our loved one. The aftershock effect of losing John may never go away completely, but Carol has learned how to move forward from the trauma of losing John, her life partner.

At the same time, I have observed surviving spouses so impacted that they experience severe depression. The point is that traumatic events happen to all of us, but feelings and responses to traumatic events differ because they occur on a continuum. And they correlate to that other "F" word—our feelings.

SO LET'S REVIEW:

Feelings, your psyche's GPS system, help to guide your behavior, mood, and overall well-being and can sneak up on you—tricky buggers.

You notice that you are feeling unusually tearful, irritable, anxious, or sad after you think you have gotten over an especially stressful period in your life. This is normal; this is aftershock.

Understand that what sparks uncomfortable feelings in one person might not be the same for the next person. It's not a competition.

As a caregiver providing psychological and emotional support to someone who is experiencing a challenging time, it is typical to feel emotionally exhausted yourself.

Recognize and acknowledge how you are feeling and give yourself permission to be kinder and gentler to yourself. Being resilient requires giving yourself grace.

CHAPTER FOUR

Aftershock Coping Skills

AFTERSHOCK, like the original trauma that caused it, can lead to unhealthy coping skills—most notably, and often the most dangerous, substance abuse. Alcohol and drugs such as the opioid OxyContin become a crutch used to numb psychological pain.

The pain itself takes many forms: anxiety, depression, feelings of guilt, shame, regret, and even self-loathing (a form of this that goes well beyond some of us mumbling "I hate myself!" while we squint into the mirror at 6 AM). People seek ways to dull or distract themselves from these uncomfortable feelings, turning to mind-numbing or mind-altering substances, a "cure" guaranteed to worsen the problem.

In this chapter, I'll help you understand and identify healthy versus unhealthy ways of coping with stress and arm you with the information necessary to make better decisions for your mental health.

Immediate Reactions to Stress

Stressful life events create responses that can contribute either positively or negatively to our self-concept—how we see ourselves. Often though, we struggle to identify how current behaviors are connected to a previous stressful event or period in our lives. The behaviors we demonstrate after a traumatic event may not become evident until weeks or even months after the event itself—this is the aftershock response.

When confronted with an especially distressing event or time in our lives, we have immediate reactions. These reactions are controlled by our brains, specifically the autonomic nervous system. Bear with me for just a moment as I wax scientific about how all this works.

The *autonomic nervous system* is a group of neurons involved in the function of various organs, such as the heart, lungs, and stomach. Within the autonomic nervous system, there are two subsystems: the *sympathetic* and *parasympathetic.*

The sympathetic nervous system can be compared to that extremely anxious friend who looks like they shoved their fork into a wall socket and were rewarded with a shock just strong enough to overstimulate them but not enough to knock them out.

Their hair is sticking straight up, pupils dilated, sweating; they have a racing heart rate and are breathless, pacing like a caged jackal, speaking so fast that you're only getting every other word they say.

This illustrates how the sympathetic nervous system empathizes with your brain's response to trauma: an immediate, visceral, physical reaction designed to prepare you for the "f****d-up" manner in which you may respond.

The second subsystem is the parasympathetic nervous system. For folks who struggle with anxiety, this system is failing them, as this subsystem is responsible for helping the body relax, which allows us to feel calm and safe.

When it is working as it should, the pupils are constricted (smaller), the heart rate is rhythmic, the breathing is slow-paced and deep, and the feel-good hormones are excreted to elevate mood.

When you think of the parasympathetic nervous system, think of that one friend who is always relaxed, lives in the moment, and says things like "Everything will work out."

And then picture yourself shaking the Zen right out of them in a pathetic attempt to relieve your own feelings of envy.

Wait. No, don't do that.

Truth be told, I could definitely use more friends who are able to successfully activate their parasympathetic nervous systems on a consistent basis. I'm betting you have picked up on the fact that I have a much closer relationship with my own sympathetic nervous system. The relationship between me and my parasympathetic nervous system has been strained for years. She is never there when I need her!

When the sympathetic nervous system is faced with a highly stressful situation, it responds in f****d-up ways. Think *freeze, fight, flight, or fawn.*

When we feel threatened, our bodies respond to our brains by urging us to reduce or escape the threat. We don't all respond in the same manner, hence the variety of f****d-up ways that are observed when we are confronted with highly stressful situations.

I. FIGHT: what I refer to as the "Mike Tyson" of stress responses. For some people, when they feel threatened, they start swinging, slapping, biting, kicking. When the FIGHT stress response is activated, the body prepares itself to react in an aggressive manner. Now, aggressiveness doesn't always equate to physical violence against another person. It can be interpreted or expressed in other ways.

If you are a prankster, you have probably instigated a FIGHT stress response multiple times. Let me give you an example.

It's bedtime in my house, and I just finished setting up the coffee for tomorrow morning. I take one final scan of the kitchen to ensure that everything is in its place. I double-check the back door to make sure it's locked. I then walk to the foyer and check the front door, making sure that it too is locked. (I watch a lot of true crime shows; don't judge me.)

I make my way upstairs. As I round the corner, my eight-year-old jumps out from behind her bedroom door and shouts, "Aaahhhhh!"

How do I respond? I scream like a banshee, swing like my life depended on it, and if I'm being completely honest, may pee a little bit (what can I say, the pelvic floor weakens after childbirth; all the moms out there know what I'm talking about!).

Now, my daughter, being no fool, has already taken off, running down the hall, turning to laugh at me as I flail my arms at the air. No real harm in this scenario, except for my wet pants.

2. FLIGHT: the stress response that says, "Run for your life!" Rather than using our fists, some of us become Usain Bolt or Florence Griffith-Joyner and hightail it out of threatening situations. The body perceives the threat or danger and provides a surge of adrenaline that courses through the bloodstream, affording the stamina and physical strength needed to run for cover and seek safety.

3. FREEZE: We've all heard the expression, "He looked like a deer in the headlights." This is a classic FREEZE stress response. Your brain might want to FIGHT or FLIGHT, but instead you FREEZE because your body believes it cannot avoid or beat the threat. Sexual assault victims will often freeze up or feel numb during an attack because they think if they just remain as still and compliant as possible, it will prevent their attacker from hurting them any further (which is sadly often true).

4. FAWN: Do you have someone in your life who's constantly apologizing for something that doesn't even warrant an apology? I went to elementary school with a girl who

would constantly apologize for what I perceived as, well, nothing. I'll give you an example: Whenever a classmate had a birthday, they would bring cupcakes in for the entire class. This girl brought in vanilla cupcakes with vanilla icing that had blue and purple sprinkles on top. Cute! And quite delicious. But as she was doling out the cupcakes, I caught her apologizing to several people. Later, I went up to her and said, "Why were you apologizing to them?" to which she replied, "I know they like chocolate cupcakes better than vanilla." I said, "You were kind enough to bring them in and share with everyone; you have nothing to be sorry about. Stop saying you are sorry when you did nothing wrong. That is so stupid." I felt like I had to protect her and help her understand that she didn't have to apologize for everything because she did nothing wrong. Granted, not the best delivery on my part. I just hope she took my harsh delivery as caring for her and not yelling at her.

Later I found out that my friend had a pretty rough home life. Her mother was an alcoholic; when drunk, she would verbally abuse my friend and make her feel like her sheer existence was a mistake. She learned at a young age that rather than fight and argue with her mother, if she simply said she was sorry, her mother would back off and move on to verbally emasculating one of her brothers.

Fawning, as you see with my childhood friend, is a stress response that is highly correlated with the residual impact of trauma that an individual may have experienced during childhood. Hence, my irrationally apologetic friend. Fawning can also present in other ways.

As I've explained, my home life was the furthest from *The Brady Bunch* you can imagine.

How did I use fawning as a protective stress response? I learned how to read the room, judge a situation, and closely observe the behavior and beliefs of the people around me, which informed how I should behave in order to avoid the conflict that would make me feel afraid, stressed, uncomfortable, or even judged by others.

Throughout my childhood, I was passed from home to home and from relative to relative during times when my parents were struggling with their own lives. I lived with my aunt and my grandmothers between three and five years old. By age fifteen, my parents were divorced, and I lived mostly with my mother. My father lived in Kensington, by then a drug-ravaged, gutted area, with a new girlfriend and infant son. My mom's addiction to heroin got so bad that we were evicted from our apartment in northeast Philadelphia. Weeks before my sophomore year of high school began, I had nowhere to live, so my cousin allowed me to live with her, her husband, and their young son in a very nice suburb of Philly.

My cousin harbored a lot of anger and pain when it came to my mother. Once very close, my mother's drug addiction had changed her and altered many of the healthy relationships she'd had with family members like my cousin. My mother said some terrible things to her. My mother wasn't much of a fighter with her fists, but boy could she tear you down with her words. And people who are addicted are master manipulators—it's a symptom of the disease. My mother's innate ability to verbally break people, mixed with her compulsion to manipulate others to get money for drugs, was like sparring with the devil herself.

Intellectually, I'm able to understand why my cousin wanted nothing to do with my mother at that time (in later years, when sober, Mom tried to make amends). But what I struggled with most was having to sit around the dinner table and listen to my cousin's husband, aunt, uncle, and other family members talk badly about my mom or even other people who struggled with addiction. After all, she was still my mother.

They had opinions, values, and beliefs different from my own. But rather than arguing with them in what I knew would be a vain attempt to get them to see things from a different perspective, I simply didn't participate in the conversation. I also worked hard to make them proud of me.

I wanted to be spared from their judgment, accepted by them, and loved because of the young lady I was becoming, not because they felt obligated to take me in or looked at me as "just another mess" of my mother's that they had to clean up. I cared too much about what they thought about everything—especially me. I worked hard to please them and kept my thoughts and feelings to myself. Just call me Queen FAWN.

Even today, as an adult, I have noticed that when confronted with an aggressive situation, I tend to respond most consistently in two f****d-up ways: FIGHTING and FAWNING. And when I look at the traumatic events I have experienced throughout my life, my instinct to respond by FIGHTING or FAWNING makes sense. Growing up, I was taught that being physical was how I should stand up for myself when confronted by a bully. Given my own parents' experiences with domestic violence, talking about our feelings was not encouraged. Screaming and punching were the "solution." As I got into my teens, I learned that there were alternatives to the FIGHT response, and I would try to implement FAWNING, although of course I didn't know that was the term for my actions.

> Given my own parents' experiences with domestic violence, talking about our feelings was not encouraged.

I can't think of a better way to illustrate these reactions than to talk about parents' (often horrible) behavior when watching their kids in sports activities.

Here's one of my own experiences.

I have two children, an eight-year-old girl and an eleven-year-old boy, both of whom play competitive basketball and soccer. Can you guess what my weekends look like? I'm pretty much an unpaid chauffeur and cheerleader. I even get to provide free therapy services to my husband, who is their coach.

During one especially entertaining soccer tournament, my son's team made it to the championship and played another team that was a year older. From my perspective, it was good practice to play an older team; it would help my son's team improve because their opponents were bigger and stronger.

As soon as the game started, parents from the opposing team started yelling, "Push him, push him!" to their players. Mind you, these kids were a year older and an average of six inches taller than our boys, who had yet to hit their growth spurt.

The first couple of times they yelled, "Push him," I barely kept my cool as the first kid being pushed was my son.

Finally, I couldn't take it any longer and blurted out, "Push him back!"

I immediately felt like a petty helicopter parent, but I could not contain myself.

The game progressed, and our team gained the lead. At that point, the doody really hit the fan, because the parents from the opposing team made their way over to our side of the field to yell, threaten, and cause a ruckus with our parents. Yes, way to set a fine example for your kids and teach them to be violent and irresponsible knuckleheads.

At first, I FAWNED. I tried to calm the situation by appeasing a dad from the other team, who had barreled over to our side of the field, yelling at a mom from our team. It took everything in me to remain composed, but it seemed to work because he retreated to his side.

Our team scored another goal. Now, normally I would be focused on cheering for the boys, but instead I found myself surveying the area for another parent from the opposing team to make an appearance. I could feel my heart pounding and my legs beginning to shake as a mom from the other team darted over to our side of the field again. She lunged at me, screaming that the goal our team scored shouldn't count for some reason or another. She was so close to me that I could smell her deodorant and identify what shade of foundation she used. With that, I put my hands up, and before I realized it, my husband was in between us—telling her to go back to her side of the field.

Next thing I know, more parents are screaming and yelling at one another, and the boys from both teams are staring at us—a total debacle.

Not one of my proudest moments as a parent, even if the other side's parents went crazy on us. But, like Dr. Winnicott says, we just have to be good enough, not even good. God knows, along with everyone else who attended that soccer tournament, I saw real proof that a threatening situation can create f****d-up responses.

Positive, Long-Term Responses to Stress

How does experiencing a traumatic or highly stressful event change you? You may not realize it, but the manner in which you approach life and view others, and even yourself, changes due to these life events you have experienced.

Many of these changes are observed in your personality and behaviors. And these behaviors help to further mold who you are—what makes you, *you!* We are often not consciously aware of these changes, and they may not be immediately recognized as being correlated to past disruptive life events, but they are.

What happens after you have gotten through a highly stressful or traumatic event? You innately try to move on and continue living.

For some folks, "living" might feel like too much, too ambitious; they merely *exist*. They continue to move through life as best they can by getting up every morning, forcing themselves out of bed, getting their kids off to school, going to work, cooking dinner, cleaning up, and finally going to bed, praying that they will be able to turn off the barrage of intrusive and anxiety-inducing thoughts that their brains play with the enthusiasm of a Metallica concert. The next day, it's rinse and repeat: same drill, different day. However, as time passes, many people rebound, start to feel or see a spark of optimism, and eventually begin living again rather than white-knuckling it through life.

When we think of the lasting effects that traumatic events can have on someone, our minds tend to naturally go toward negative responses, such as depression, anxiety, irritability, sleep disturbances, and feelings of worthlessness and guilt, just to name a few. However, there are also positive residual effects born out of highly stressful events that we tend to focus less on. I want to introduce you to the *upside* of aftershock, a delayed trauma response that is overlooked because we tend to dedicate all our energy to what we perceive to be the "bad" parts of ourselves.

I am reminded of a quote from a play by William Shakespeare: "The evil that men do lives after them; the good is oft interred with their bones." Another quote from Imam al-Shafi'i Rahimullah also comes to mind: "If you do ninety-nine things correct, and one thing incorrect, people will ignore the ninety-nine, and spread the one mistake." These quotes speak to how we treat ourselves. Many of us zero in on the negative parts of ourselves and become our own worst critic. We often neglect the good parts of ourselves that are realized as a result of the adversity or trauma we encounter.

Post-Traumatic Growth: The Silver Lining

Time to introduce you to two more brilliant psychologists: Richard Tedeschi, PhD,[8] and Lawrence Calhoun, PhD, the theorists who came up with the concept of post-traumatic growth (PTG).

PTG is a theory that posits that people who have withstood highly distressing or traumatic events may experience positive psychological changes as a result of the adversity they endured.

When faced with adversity, we have the psychological tools to work through it. Remember, working through it does not mean that we won't fail. We'll endure bumps, scrapes, and bruises to our psyches; this is normal—even expected. Remember, life isn't supposed to be easy. Pain is part of the human experience. How we manage the pain is what leads to psychological growth. How we react and respond to distressful life events can be up to us.

Prior to pursuing my doctoral degree in clinical psychology, I worked in media sales. I worked for AccuWeather.com, selling online advertisements across the country. During my time at

AccuWeather I had the privilege of working with some amazing people. At the time, I knew I liked the people I worked with because they made the grind of a highly competitive sales gig bearable. But it was after I left the industry and grew as a person that I *really* came to appreciate them.

In sales, your ego takes a beating because no matter how fantastic a product you may be selling, most prospects are not ready to buy. When people tell you "No" a gazillion times a day, you begin to take it personally, no matter how many times you tell yourself that this is simply the nature of the profession. Intellectually, you know that the rejection isn't personal, but at the end of the day in the "wonderful world of sales," you are only as good as your last successful month of crushing your sales goal. Life in sales is the proverbial roller-coaster ride. One month you're the queen; the next month, a lowly scullery maid if you fail to meet your goal.

Life in sales is the proverbial roller-coaster ride.

My coworker buddy Jason had the gift of making us all laugh when we felt like the lowly servants. From wrapping my entire desk in Christmas wrapping paper to quietly mocking upper management like John Krasinski's character, Jim, from the hit television show *The Office*, Jason used humor to help us get through those challenging months when sales were dismal. And we all benefited from it.

Another coworker, Eric, was initially hired to sell advertising for AccuWeather.com on mobile devices. Now, this was well over a decade ago, so Eric was tasked with simultaneously educating clients on a novel form of advertising and convincing them to invest their money with AccuWeather.com on this progressive advertising approach. If I'm being completely honest, we all felt bad for Eric because his job was the toughest, and he knew it.

One day, Eric, Jason, and I were commiserating about sales, and Eric said something that stuck with me. He was talking about a sale that he thought he was on the brink of closing. Keep in mind that if we heard the word "no" twenty times a day, Eric heard it sixty times. It was the nature of what he was selling—something new and not yet understood by our clients—that made it so difficult and had nothing to do with his ability as a salesperson.

Despite all the pressure that Eric felt to make a sale, he demonstrated admirable composure, which says a lot about his character. What resonated with me was something that he said during our conversation. He said, "I did everything I could. I developed a concise and thoughtful presentation. Listened to the clients' concerns and answered their questions. I am cautiously optimistic that I will make this sale." Thus, Eric taught me about *cautious optimism*. Despite getting his ego beaten up on a daily basis, mixed with the constant fear of losing his job for not meeting his sales goals, he proceeded with cautious optimism—a glass half-full mentality that can serve us all well.

Eric learned how to proceed with cautious optimism rather than total nihilism or defeat. It would have been easy for him to take a negativistic approach, blame the product, the company, and even himself for his lack of sales. Instead, he chose to exercise his psychological/emotional IQ, assess the situation, and find a way to get through it rather than succumb to it. Like Eric, we all have the ability to remain hopeful and encouraging despite some terrible life circumstances that have been thrown in our path. Hopefulness is not to be confused with naïveté.

Just look at Philly's most beloved underdog (next to the Philadelphia Eagles—E-A-G-L-E-S!), Rocky Balboa. Rocky's motivation to win is constantly undermined. He is bullied, put down, and beaten to a pulp in all six *Rocky* movies. And every time, he refuses to give up. That said his relentless belief in himself makes him resilient.

Resilience is a positive attribute that comes out of having gone through a particularly stressful time in life. Like the Japanese proverb from Naoki Higashida, "Fall down seven times, get up eight," people who are resilient, like Rocky, look at falling as an opportunity to learn. Was he frustrated? Yes! Did he sulk for a bit? Absolutely. But he also took a step back and reassessed how he could learn from each and every one of his falls. Humility, tenacity, a healthy self-concept and worldview, and humor are some of the possible positive, long-term responses to getting knocked down (trauma) that Rocky adopted. These key ingredients are considered healthy forms of coping, and we can all do well to emulate Rocky's innate coping skills.

There are five domains or, shall we say, upsides identified through post-traumatic growth. Drum roll please . . .

1. A deeper respect and appreciation for life;
2. The ability to develop closer, meaningful relationships;

3. Openness to new possibilities;

4. Spiritual development; and

5. Greater resilience through adversity.

The best way to see these five domains come to life is through actual stories from others' lives. Shall we?

JAMAL

I completed my postdoctoral fellowship in a community mental health clinic. During my time there, I had the privilege of working with a broad range of patients of various races, cultures, socioeconomic statuses, sexual orientations, and gender identities with a wide range of various mental health concerns that humans everywhere struggle with. I remember many of the people I worked with, as I learned so much from them, even though I was the one trained to help them learn how to manage their mental health. But when it comes to the subject of post-traumatic growth, one person comes immediately to mind: Jamal.

Jamal was in his midforties and was referred to me for anxiety. I learned that he was a single dad of two young girls. His youngest girl was in eighth grade, and his older girl was in her freshman year at a local high school that was well-known for its highly competitive athletic programs. Jamal told me that when his girls were toddlers, he lost his wife in a tragic car accident. She was driving home from a business trip, got hit by an eighteen-wheeler, and was ejected from her car. She was found about fifty feet away from the vehicle and pronounced dead at the scene of the accident. What a horror!

Prior to his wife's tragic death, Jamal was an architect and traveled into the city daily from a surrounding suburb. However, after his wife's death, he stopped and dedicated himself to raising his daughters. Jamal had four siblings, all of whom rallied around him and his daughters after the accident. He came from a close-knit family that consistently demonstrated love and support for Jamal and his daughters.

Fast-forward to ten years later, and Jamal was in my office because he was suffering with anxiety.

During our first few sessions, I spent most of the time listening to Jamal and getting to learn more about him. He felt compelled to tell me that he had accepted his wife's untimely death. With that, I knew that it was not a topic that he was ready to discuss. I respected his wishes. Rule number one as a therapist: It is imperative to meet your patients or clients where they are. Follow their lead and walk alongside them, not in front of them. In order for Jamal to trust me with his most private and painful feelings, I had to earn his trust. Jamal wanted to talk about his anxiety because it was preventing him from going back to work full-time. So that's what we did. We dug into why he felt anxious and discovered that his girls were older and didn't need him as much as they had when they were younger. They were becoming more independent. And for the first time in ten years, Jamal had the opportunity to do something he hadn't done in a long time: FEEL.

With his daughters getting older and growing independent, they also began to socialize more and hang out with their friends, which meant that Jamal had more time to himself. His anxiety was rooted in the unknown, the uncertainty that accompanied this next phase of life. He knew he no longer wanted to work as an architect but was unsure of what he wanted to do. He gave his daughters the autonomy they needed to develop a healthy independence and social life, but he worried about them. His worry was more than that of a typical parent of a teenager, largely due to the unexpected passing of his wife. He didn't want anything bad to happen to his girls. They were more independent, which meant that he could not protect them in the same way he had when they were little. This constant worry created feelings of severe anxiety for Jamal, who perhaps felt guilty that he hadn't been able protect his wife.

Finally, after several months of therapy, he talked about his wife in a very different way than he had initially. What made it different was that his words were accompanied by *emotion*. He let it out. After ten years of holding his emotions in and keeping it together for his daughters, Jamal allowed himself to feel, to cry, to grieve his wife. I felt privileged that he allowed me to witness his vulnerability. It takes a lot to share your most protected feelings and emotions. Jamal had a major breakthrough. He probably felt like he was emotionally placed on display for me and others to judge harshly. However, as he continued to progress in therapy, his belief and confidence in himself continued to grow.

> It takes a lot to share your most protected feelings and emotions.

One day, Jamal came to therapy noticeably anxious. This was not typical as he always did a good job of masking his anxiety. He explained that he had been asked to be the athletic director at the high school his daughter attended. This particular school was well-known and highly regarded for its athletic programs: football, basketball, baseball, softball, lacrosse, and track. It was a high-profile job, and Jamal was the perfect candidate.

During the session, he expressed his fear of possibly failing. At this point in the therapeutic relationship, I felt that I had a good understanding of Jamal. I knew he was more than capable. I offered him some much-needed reassurance and allowed him the time and space to make his decision.

It just so happened that my postdoctoral fellowship was coming to an end. Jamal and I had only a few sessions left. During one of our last sessions, he shared with me that he had attended a meeting with the school principal and with the current athletic director, who was looking forward to retiring and passing the torch to Jamal. Jamal proposed that the current athletic director stay one more year to show him the ropes, and she agreed to his proposal. Jamal and I had another session or two after sharing this excellent news, and then we parted ways.

Fast-forward six years, and my husband took my children to a basketball camp at the high school where Jamal had been slated to be the athletic director. Therapists do not disclose information about their clients. We do not break confidentiality unless the client is considering or endorsing suicidal and/or homicidal ideation and/or intent, or if it is discovered that a child's safety is at risk during a session with a client.

Point being that my husband does not know who I treat. Jamal was working the basketball camp and started chatting with my husband at parent drop-off. He noticed my husband's last name and asked if he knew me. To which my husband replied, "Geri-Lynn is my wife."

Jamal then disclosed to my husband that I treated him in therapy. So my husband said, "Do you wanna say hi to her?"

I answered the phone thinking it was my husband, but then I heard Jamal's voice on the other end. I nearly fell over when I heard, "What's up, doc, it's your favorite patient!"

He shared with me that he was the athletic director and that he and his daughters were doing great! I was overwhelmed with happiness for Jamal. He went on to tell me how much I helped him, which may be true—at least I would like to think so. From my perspective, Jamal helped me become a better therapist.

Jamal's story is a real-life depiction of what post-traumatic growth looks like. The pain of losing your partner is devastating at any age, let alone when your children are toddlers. The aftershock of Jamal losing his wife extended years. He came into therapy for anxiety a decade after her death, not realizing that the root of his anxiety was connected to unresolved, prolonged grief.

For many folks, post-traumatic growth can occur without any formal intervention or therapy. Jamal made many meaningful strides on his own regarding his ability to function, raise his girls, and navigate a new world that did not include his life partner. However, as his girls grew up and became more independent, feelings of grief that he had pushed down to be present for his daughters floated back up to the surface in the form of anxiety. Therapy afforded Jamal the opportunity to address his anxiety, which paved the way for him to finally work on the feelings of loss he had experienced after his wife's untimely death.

Today, he moves through life with a deeper appreciation for every day, grateful to be present for his daughters. The bond he has nurtured with them is one that he will forever cherish. Jamal also possesses the understanding and humility that life is not guaranteed. He has allowed himself to be vulnerable by accepting love and emotional support from his siblings, parents, in-laws, and close friends, which ultimately helped him develop deeper, more meaningful relationships with the people in his life. He had been raised Catholic, and rather than straying away from his faith, he leaned into it after his wife died. Of course, he was initially angry at his God for what he perceived as the creation of pain and suffering for him and his daughters. But as time passed, he used his faith as a means of coping—for hope. He shared with me that even though we hadn't worked together for six years, he still prayed for me and my family.

It has given me such joy to witness Jamal, who once doubted his ability due to his anxiety, become the athletic director of a school that has highly competitive athletic programs. A true inspiration, Jamal's post-traumatic growth was born out of his belief in himself in the face of adversity. Rather than succumbing to his mental health concerns, he took the first step by reaching out for help, which is demonstrative of resilience. Rocky Balboa would be proud!

Negative Long-Term Responses to Stress

Let's be real. Sometimes when life throws us lemons, we say, "Screw making lemonade, I'd rather throw ninety-mile-an-hour fastballs at the heads of everyone who has made life seem like a constant shit show with no final episode in sight!" I know all of you have thought about this. You might not have ever said it out loud, but you definitely thought about it. And if you're from Philly, like I am, we don't hold back from sharing how we feel. And guess what. It feels good to say it, to get it out. In fact, I'll go so far as to say that it is actually therapeutic to express our thoughts and feelings rather than stuffing them down, holding them in, and neglecting how they might impact our moods and self-concept.

Here's the thing: Saying how you feel is only one part of the magic formula needed to help us better manage our mental health when terrible things happen to us. Oftentimes, we subconsciously lean on things like food, alcohol, and drugs to improve our mood or stop us from experiencing painful feelings altogether. We pick up unhealthy coping strategies that might not be apparent to us at first. However, as time progresses, we realize that the very thing we were leaning on to help us feel better, feel less, or not feel anything at all has created more havoc and heartbreak in our lives.

According to the Centers for Disease Control,[9] over half the United States population will receive a mental illness diagnosis. Now, after reading this statistic, keep these two important pieces of information in mind: (1) That number only represents individuals who have *sought* help for their mental health; (2) Think of all the people who have not felt comfortable enough to seek mental health treatment due to stigma, lack of access to treatment, and/or lack of finances or insurance to secure treatment.

So the CDC's statistic is not, strictly speaking, a reliable figure because there are so many folks who have not been identified and diagnosed. Some people will simply refuse treatment for a number of reasons while for many folks, it can take years before they get to the point where they realize they need mental health support.

LAUREN

I remember the first time I met Lauren. I was barely twenty-three years old, naively wide-eyed, and ready to start my career slinging thirty- and sixty-second radio spots for one of Philadelphia's top 40 radio stations. My first day at this new gig, I was introduced to Lauren. She had that fresh-faced, natural beauty thing going for her—shoulder-length, sandy blond hair, striking blue eyes. Lauren dressed to the nines and was very well-spoken. She was about ten years older than me. I was happy to be sharing an office with her because I was able to learn the tricks of the trade from someone far more experienced.

I listened to how she pitched potential clients, negotiated rates, and carried herself in an office predominantly made up of male colleagues. She was engaging, but like many seasoned sales representatives in media, Lauren was probably thinking that I wouldn't be her office mate for long. There is a saying that one of my mentors, "Fletch," shared with me when I landed my first radio gig—"Radio—it eats its young." I guess that was Fletch's way of inspiring me.

Days turned into weeks, and weeks turned into my first year in radio sales. If you can last a year, you have "officially" made it in radio. By then, Lauren figured I wasn't going anywhere, and we started to hang out more after work. I learned that Lauren was divorced with two daughters. Her oldest daughter was in second grade, and her little one was in kindergarten.

As time went on, she grew more comfortable talking with me about her family situation. She would have some pretty heated phone calls with her former husband, Bruce, when I was within earshot. This was drastically different from my first six months in the office, when she would take calls with Bruce in an empty conference room. The level of ease we felt around each other was reflective of our growing friendship.

Lauren and Bruce shared joint custody of their two young children. They lived close enough to each other that their children could remain in the same school district. This also allowed them to alternate weeks—living with Lauren for one week, then Bruce for the next. It appeared to be a sensible arrangement, at least as sensible as it could be when shuttling children from parent to parent.

One night Lauren and I grabbed a drink after work, and she began to share more with me about Bruce and the reason for their divorce. She explained that he was controlling about everything— how Lauren looked, what she wore, what she ate, the friends she chose, his desire to not have her work, how they made love—the list seemed endless. It got to the point where Lauren got very depressed. She felt alone and isolated from everyone she loved.

Near the end of her marriage and throughout her divorce, she began to drink. At first, she would drink only a glass or two of wine at night because it helped her fall asleep. However, as divorce proceedings progressed, and Bruce grew more disdainful toward Lauren, one or two glasses of wine a night increased to a bottle.

The more that Lauren and I hung out after work, the more I began to notice how much she drank. Now, don't get me wrong. In my early twenties, I knew how to have a good time. But I also knew when to call it a night. Lauren was a different story.

One night, after a work event, a group of us decided to keep the momentum going by checking out a new lounge that had opened in Center City, Philadelphia. As the party was winding down, I noticed that Lauren was nowhere to be found. I and a few other folks from the office found Lauren's car in the parking lot but no Lauren. I must have called her cell phone a hundred times before an unknown, deep voice picked up and said, "Hey, I've been telling your friend to pick up the phone." It turns out Lauren left the lounge with a handsome face she had met a couple of hours earlier in the evening. Handsome Face put Lauren on the phone with me, and I encouraged her to meet us in the parking lot so we could drive her home. I also asked if I could come pick her up from this handsome stranger's apartment, to which she replied by giggling and hanging up on me.

The weekend passed, and I didn't hear from Lauren, but given my past experiences with her, I was pretty certain she had made it home safely. Monday morning rolled around, and my worry skyrocketed because I didn't see her when I arrived at the office. I kept looking at the clock: 8:30 AM, 8:41 AM, 8:55 AM. Every minute felt like an hour. Finally, Lauren walked into our office. She had her hair pulled back into a clip, no makeup on, and a coffee thermos. She greeted me with "Good morning, Ger" like she always did and proceeded to her desk to put on her face. It appeared to be business as usual, but the longer Lauren and I worked together, the more obvious it became that she had a problem.

I worked with Lauren for three years before moving on to my next gig. The last year we worked together, it became even more apparent that Lauren was struggling with her drinking. So much so that she started putting vodka in her coffee thermos every morning as if to take the edge off from drinking too much the night prior. Her work began to suffer, and so did her relationship with her family.

About six months after I started working at another radio station, Lauren called me. She had finally had enough and wanted to get treatment for her drinking. I encouraged her to get the help she needed and let her know how happy I was that she was taking such a huge step toward her recovery. Lauren was accepted into an inpatient rehabilitation program where she was treated for alcohol use disorder. Nearly fifteen years later, she continues to work on her recovery.

Lauren's story demonstrates how going through a tough time, like a nasty divorce, can lead to some unhealthy coping skills. The stress of the divorce made it difficult for her to sleep, so she began to use wine as her sleep aid. It did not occur to Lauren that her behavior could lead to an alcohol use disorder. The more distressed Lauren felt, the more she drank.

Like Lauren, folks abuse alcohol, drugs, or food as a way to numb themselves from psychological pain. My dear friend Jerry, who is six years sober, explained it best by saying, "It's the time outside of yourself that is addicting." Abusing alcohol gave Lauren a respite, a break from her thoughts, feelings, and emotions. But here's the thing: That temporary break is just that—temporary and short-lived. And what makes it even more complicated are the additional problems and stress that abusing alcohol caused Lauren. She lost several good-paying media sales jobs because her drinking impeded her performance. Lauren's children did not want to spend time with her because she acted differently around them when she drank.

> The funny thing about unhealthy coping skills is that we are initially oblivious to our own unhealthy behaviors.

The funny thing about unhealthy coping skills is that we are initially oblivious to our own unhealthy behaviors. Did Lauren plan on abusing alcohol as a way to manage the trauma and stress of her divorce? Absolutely not! We are too close to ourselves and our internal monologue (which is often cloaked in delusion) to recognize when we're too far down the rabbit hole. When we do finally scratch and claw our way back to the surface, we're faced with the consequences of the behaviors we demonstrated in active addiction. For Lauren, her alcohol abuse caused more problems for her, on top of an already tumultuous divorce. And this is pretty much always the case.

So, finally, Lauren did recognize that her alcohol abuse was affecting her relationships, her career, and how she felt about herself. She wanted to make a change. And despite all the fear and anxiety involved in seeking help, Lauren did it. What many folks don't realize is that making the decision to get help is scary. Even though drinking was ruining Lauren's life, she felt a level of comfort by continuing to do it; it was the "devil she knows."

While seeking treatment for drinking would ultimately change her life for the better, it was uncharted territory for Lauren. She would be exchanging a coping skill, albeit an unhealthy one, for treatment that would make her vulnerable to feeling again—something that she worked so hard to escape by drinking. Even though she was anxious and fearful about seeking treatment for her drinking, she did not let it stop her. Her drive to push forward and face all her feelings head-on speaks to her resilience. Like Jamal, Lauren was able to experience positive change through a chaotic divorce and alcohol abuse, which demonstrates post-traumatic growth—the silver lining.

SO LET'S REVIEW:

The mind and body connection are powerful. When we feel threatened, our autonomic nervous system, composed of the sympathetic and parasympathetic nervous systems, rises to the occasion to help us.

We respond in f****d-up ways such as freeze, fight, flight, and fawn.

Remember PTG (post-traumatic growth)—people (like you and me) who have experienced highly distressed situations can experience positive psychological changes from the adversity they endured.

A few of the positive long-term effects that are born out of aftershock are humility, tenacity, cautious optimism, and humor.

CHAPTER FIVE

Symptoms of Aftershock and the Need for Self-Care

BEFORE WE TALK about how to care for yourself when aftershock hits, it's important to learn how to recognize after-shock trauma symptoms. Once you learn how to recognize them, you can help yourself deal and heal.

First, have you had any of these issues lately?

- Fatigue;
- Lack of energy;
- No interest in activities or social gatherings that once gave you joy;
- Irritability;

- Feeling bad about yourself or feeling worthless ("Why am I such a piece of...");
- Finding it difficult to do even the simplest things in life, like getting out of bed, showering, straightening up the house, taking your kid to soccer practice, or cooking; and
- Of course, let's not forget anxiety— my personal favorite.

Let me count the ways that I can worry about *anything*. It's like my brain plays this screwed-up game in my head called "What If?" What if the email I sent my boss is misconstrued? What if she takes it the wrong way and fires me? What if my husband and son get into a horrific car accident on their way to a soccer tournament because I should have driven? What if the performance I have been practicing for the past month ends up being horrible or, once the curtain opens, I freeze and forget my lines? What if the deodorant I am using causes breast cancer because there is aluminum in it . . . what if . . . *what if . . . what if?!*

The list goes on and on, and it includes clinical depression, which is an overwhelming feeling of emptiness and apathy when your ability to feel happy or even sad atrophies. You just exist. You don't feel like you're *living,* merely taking up space.

Our symptoms can be triggered by our internal monologues and the way we talk to ourselves. That little voice inside our heads can be very cruel.

I know I'm dating myself here, but I'm reminded of a hit song by a 1990s band called Lit: "My Own Worst Enemy." That is exactly what our internal monologue is—an enemy. What we say to and about ourselves is sometimes more damaging than the feedback we receive from others. I have shared this perspective with a client I worked with named Nicole. Nicole began participating in therapy with me because she was highly anxious. Together, we learned that Nicole possessed a very poor self-concept. Growing up, Nicole was made to feel that nothing she did was good enough by her caregivers. She was often criticized for everything, from the romantic partners she chose to the clothes she wore, if they did not align with her family's ideals. Nicole was made to feel less than because she was different from her family origin, which impacted how she viewed herself. She believed she was "damaged goods," which instigated feelings of severe anxiety due to internalized feelings of inferiority.

Self-Care for Aftershock

So what is the answer? How can you learn to manage these emotions and change the dirge in your head to a victory march?

Recognize what's happening, and consciously work to override it. Tell that gloomy deadbeat that lives rent free in your brain to stick a sock in it, or better yet teach her (and by *her*, I mean *you*) to be more self-compassionate.

Realize and admit the obvious: The useless things that you play on a loop in your head, adding in the echoing commentary of others, all validating what a rotten person you are, *are not helpful.* Give yourself credit. Stop judging yourself more harshly than you would others.

Here are some ideas that will help you deal with aftershock symptoms.

Self-Compassion

What do I mean by self-compassion?

I define it thus: the desire and ability to feel motivated to relieve yourself from psychological pain and suffering.

That is, give yourself grace. So often we focus on our imperfections, the aspects or traits in ourselves that we don't like and wish we could cut off or change. We play the loser in our narrative. We are that school-age bully, constantly putting ourselves down.

If you wish to navigate through life without constantly feeling depressed and anxious, a priceless skill you can develop is to be kinder and more forgiving to yourself. This means making a sea change in the way you evaluate and determine your own self-worth.

The first step is learning how to love yourself. I know this might sound a little too woo-woo, but trust me. And *love yourself unconditionally, not contingently.*

Using myself as an example, I am terrible at giving myself permission to relax and just be, primarily because I equate my own self-worth with my accomplishments. And if I'm not crushing the goals I set out for myself, my ability to demonstrate self-compassion fades to black.

Loving yourself starts with *acceptance.*

As they say, "It is what it is." In my case, in the past, when I'd throw my hands in the air and mutter this expression aloud, it would be out of the disappointment that came with not being able to change something or someone. When I use this expression today, it's not to express disappointment but acceptance. I'm learning how to accept the fact that some of the emotions I experience in life are going to be uncomfortable, sad, aggravating, even nerve-wracking (the list goes on). And that's okay!

The COVID-19 pandemic provided an opportunity to learn acceptance. It's okay for you not to feel okay. Acknowledge that there will be times when things happen that are out of your control and that these things can cause pain.

When we experience psychological pain, learning how to sit with it—that *it is what it is*—can offer relief (being okay with not being okay) and pave the way for a change of perspective.

The goal is to recognize how you feel, accept it, and try to work through it, not around it.

Supportive Connections

Here is one of my favorite pieces of advice and something I believe we often overlook: Make connections with people who are supports, not life suckers. Surround yourself with people who will give you grace—that thing you so often deny yourself.

When you feel down and at your worst, the last thing you need is for a family member or "friend" to rub salt in your wounds. Yes, you are your own worst enemy. However, some family and friends are more than willing to compete for that title.

Talking with friends, aka life givers, who will support a venting session or remind me that my internal monologue is a nasty gossip has helped to maintain what is left of my sanity. I was talking to a physician friend of mine who had studied Judaism. During one of our conversations, which almost always consisted of how we might help a patient, I asked him, "How do you treat yourself, or what do you say to yourself when you mess up or feel bad?"

"Rabbi Hillel, one of the greatest Jewish philosophers of all time, had a great saying that has helped me during tough times. He said, 'If I am not for myself, who will be for me? If I am not for others, what am I? And if not now, when?'" he answered.

After we spoke, I immediately did a Google search for the quote by Rabbi Hillel, wrote it down on a sticky note, and stuck it on my computer. Now, every time I start to turn on myself, I read Rabbi Hillel's quote, take four deep breaths, and give myself permission to:

- Duct-tape shut the big mouth on that little Geri-Lynn in my head;
- Be my own cheerleader; and
- Move forward.

Try it yourself! Jot down the Rabbi's wise words and create your own three-step process to help change that voice in your head from harsh and critical to kind and empowering.

Mis-Connections: Social Media Can Be Such an Isolating Place

It's not just your envious "friends" and misanthropic relatives that can sabotage you. It's those distant, anonymous trolls on the web who tell you how great they are and what a useless nothing you are. Data is piling up that too much social media makes us feel like crap about ourselves. So if you resemble that remark, cut back! Decrease your screen time—shut this down, even if it is just for an hour or two. We have access to so much information on our phones, from social media platforms like Twitter and TikTok to news feeds. We get hit with a constant flow of information based on our scrolling habits, which sucks us in for even longer.

As for TikTok, I didn't know what the hell it was until my kids downloaded it on my phone so they could make videos. Before I knew it, I was stuck in a TikTok hostage situation in which I couldn't stop watching videos of people lip-syncing lines from movies and making meals that I would never even have imagined, much less attempted, before watching. The stimulation and access to information often ended with me feeling more anxious, or at least dull-witted and blah.

So I promised myself to limit my time scrolling social-media platforms, after-hours work e-mails, and carrying my phone around, because simply having it on me made it easy to work and scroll more—and more is not always better.

Do Something for You

Hey, in addition to getting your inner voice on your side, how about trying this: *do one thing every day that makes you happy and is just for you.*

If you enjoy taking a bath, playing tennis, or even watching trashy reality TV, make time to do it daily. Make your happiness a priority; even if it's just for a few minutes, it can go a long way.

Move Your Ass!

Yogi Berra is reported to have said about baseball: "Ninety percent of this game is half mental."

I suppose he knew what he meant.

But I will flip this "Yogi-ism" paradox to: *"Ninety percent of mental health is half physical."*

Confused?

That's just my Yogi way of saying that exercise and physical health support your mental health.

I know there are a number of us out there who cringe at the thought of having to exercise, myself included. But if I have learned one thing about exercise, it's that I feel so much better after I finish. That dopamine rush that is released after exercise helps to modulate your mood for the better.

Dopamine is known as the feel-good neurotransmitter because it's correlated to pleasure. And, for the record, when I say exercise, I don't mean running a 10K if you've never run a day in your life, or bench-pressing 200 pounds if you've never picked up a free weight. Literally, one step at a time!

> Going for a thirty- to forty-five-minute walk daily will benefit both your body and your brain.

Going for a thirty- to forty-five-minute walk daily will benefit both your body and your brain. And if you can do it outside, even better. I started walking daily at the start of the pandemic and haven't stopped. Time outside alone has also helped me a lot. My daily walks have saved my husband's and kids' lives ten times over!

Laugh at Yourself and Lean on Friends

During my doctoral program, I learned to take myself less seriously. Believe me, competitive academic programs don't often lend themselves to the concept of humor as a coping skill.

In the beginning, I constantly looked around the classrooms and found myself wondering if I even deserved a seat at the table. I worked hard to perform well academically and worked even harder to keep it together.

You would think that a group of aspiring clinical psychologists would be supportive and nonjudgmental of one another, but that intention gets lost on so many of us because of our inability to abandon unrealistic expectations of ourselves. So, during that time, as I learned how to be my own best friend, I would say to myself, *It isn't about striving for perfect grades; it's about soaking up all the knowledge I can, trying my best, and learning to live with whatever comes out of the experience.*

Those pep talks were in addition to the support I got from my best friend. Sue is a life giver, and she helped me learn how to laugh when things felt overwhelming. I would share my fears or self-doubts with Sue (a registered nurse), and she always did a great job of mocking me and reminding me who I was and that I could handle it. Like when I was going for my doctorate.

I said to her one evening over a glass of box wine, "I can't freakin' do this! I can't compete with these brainiac, silver-spoon types. Maybe I'm not cut out for this doctor thing!"

Sue's kind words saved me. Well, first she said, "Oh, shut *up*! When did you start doubting yourself? This is not the Geri-Lynn

I know." Then she said, "You are one of the most driven people I have ever met, and you are gonna crush this thing. Even if you fall on your ass a few times, you'll get up, I'll slap you around, and you'll try again. And you *will* do this!"

She was right. My internal monologue shifted and became more encouraging, and my conversations with Sue got longer!

So step back and laugh at yourself at times, and tell your *real* friends to give you an elbow when you're taking yourself so seriously that you are damaging your own well-being.

Pay It Forward

Reward is a two-way street when it comes to paying it forward. The recipient of a random act of kindness feels appreciated, cared for, worthy, and loved. The person being kind feels happy because they helped someone else. A win–win.

I live right outside Philly, and if you know anything about the area, Dunkin' Donuts is the lifeblood that keeps us going. Every now and then, I will pay for the coffee of the person behind me in the Dunkin' Donuts drive-through. I know this might sound strange, but that small gesture can make the day of someone who is struggling to keep it together. Just knowing that I did something nice for someone else makes me feel good.

Acts of kindness need not be monetary or caffeinated; they can be compliments. My younger sister, Dominique, excels at making people feel good about themselves in a genuine way. She works for a large OB-GYN practice. All day long, she sees pregnant women. And if you know anything about the various stages of pregnancy, you know there are times when you feel as though your body is being invaded by a six- to ten-pound creature (well, it actually *is*) whose main purpose is to make your body morph into an unrecognizable lump of yourself. Let's just say that your self-esteem will have seen better days.

Dominique has the talent of making these women feel good about themselves, if even for a few minutes, by complimenting their curves and injecting them with much-needed hope that they will be kick-ass moms equipped to handle whatever their baby throws at them (literally and figuratively). When I talked to Dominique about her talent, she said with a glowing smile, "It makes me feel good to make my patients feel good about themselves."

What more could we want?

Spend time today and every day helping others cope and feel good about themselves. Let's be here for one another.

Reflect on Your Position in Life Without Comparing Yourself to Others

We are notorious for comparing ourselves to other people who we believe "have it all"—the best partner, nicest house, toniest zip code, most enviable career, hottest body, most exotic car, you name it! And envy is one ugly emotion. It can even lead us to hate others.

But who's at fault here, them or us?

Simple: it's us, for putting them on a pedestal and lusting after the life we think they have and that we convince ourselves we want.

Yet, there is no real fault here; it's human to compare yourself. But, like anything in life, balance is essential. If you're feeling bad about yourself, it's time to superglue that unhelpful internal monologue shut.

If you're feeling bad about yourself, it's time to superglue that unhelpful internal monologue shut.

It's that little dictator in your head again, saying, *Look at her! She has her dream job, two beautiful children, and abs for days.* Meanwhile, you've given up on your dream of becoming a business owner, your kids don't even talk to you at the moment, and you haven't been able to get rid of your muffin top, no matter how much you try.

What to do? Reel in that harsh inner voice. Replace the envy monster with a flattery fairy who reminds you how much you have and how far you've come, who tells you that others might not have *quite* the perfect lives they show on Insta.

The next time you get sucked into a self-deprecating social media scroll of 900 of your "closest friends," who only present the best of themselves to the public, STOP. Take a moment to think of a list of three positive traits about yourself.

Okay, I'll go first: I have great hair, I am a good listener, and I am a bad-ass bitch!

Now, your turn!

Yep! Be Kind to Yourself!

Learn to recognize the aftershock symptoms of anxiety and depression. Get help from others, either from understanding buddies or from healthcare professionals.

But start with yourself.

Listen, it's important that you learn to take care of yourself, that you treat yourself kindly, that you don't bash yourself mercilessly in ways that you would never bash your friends or family. I mean it. Think about it the next time you're in the middle of self-flagellation: Would you do that to your best friend? If your best friend came to you with a problem, would you hack on her, degrade her, call her the same kind of names you call yourself?

I doubt it. Or you wouldn't have many friends.

Stop being your own worst enemy in time to become your own best friend. That's important for you, and it's a support for those you love. We learn from flying on airlines that if the oxygen masks drop, we should put on our own masks first. That just means, if we can't breathe, we can't help anyone else. That applies to our everyday lives. If you don't give yourself breathing room, you won't do anyone any good.

Be kind to yourself. Prop up your own damaged ego. Remind yourself of what you have accomplished and what you plan to accomplish. Make yourself feel good about yourself, which will, in turn, make you better at making others feel good.

Life is tough. Don't make it tougher. Make it more fun, sweeter, and less stressful. You got this!

SO LET'S REVIEW:

The internal monologue, aka the little dictator that lives rent free in your head, can be your own worst enemy. Slap some duct tape on their mouth and show yourself some love by writing or saying out loud three things you like about yourself.

Loving yourself starts with accepting who you are, which includes the good and the bad parts of yourself.

Surround yourself with life givers, not life suckers.

Therapy is a resource you can tap into to help you navigate through life when you feel overwhelmed. There is no shame in the therapy game, my friends!

Do one thing every day that puts a smile on your face. It can be as simple as indulging in your favorite latte, watching your favorite television show, or paying it forward by helping someone else out.

Get up, get out, and get moving. Taking a thirty-minute walk can do wonders for your mental health.

Remember the irony in how isolating so-called "social" media can be. If you notice that you are feeling drained, anxious, or just blah after being on social media, put the screen down, take a break.

Comparing yourself to others' social media posts can be likened to the bright lights being turned on in a bar/nightclub at last call when you realize the hottie you thought you were dancing with all night is, well, not so hot, LOL!

CHAPTER SIX

The Stigma of Mental Illness and Accompanying Treatments

WHY IS IT THAT WE WILL HURRY to seek treatment for physical ailments but hesitate to get help for emotional issues?

The answer is complicated, so let's explore the issues that may prevent you from getting help. First, let me share this with you: I'm a psychologist, trained in helping people who struggle with an array of mental health concerns ranging from trauma to anxiety to drug and alcohol abuse. I find myself reaching out for mental health treatment at times because I too get overwhelmed with the stress of life.

Let me be straight up with you: The stigma surrounding seeking help for mental health concerns is maddening. Please do not allow other people's ignorance to persuade you from reaching out for help from a mental health professional. It is your business. You are not obligated to disclose treatment you are getting for your mental health in the same way you do not announce that you're getting your annual mammogram or prostate exam.

Stigma. The word itself sounds cringy and off-putting. It is derived from an ancient Greek term meaning "to mark as a sign of shame, punishment, or disgrace." Think of the classic novel *The Scarlet Letter.* As you know, Hester Prynne, the main character in the Nathaniel Hawthorne story, is a young woman ostracized by her community for committing adultery and having a child out of wedlock. As punishment, she is charged with wearing a large red letter "A" on her clothing—her *stigma*—as a constant reminder to herself and the community at large of the moral sin she committed. The letter sewn onto Hester's clothing creates an environment in which she is scorned and mocked by members of the community. Yet, despite all the harassment Hester suffers, she remains compassionate and dignified. Her resilience and self-belief eventually quiets those who continuously spoke badly about her. We can learn from this that the stigma placed upon her was unjust and that we can stand apart from unjust stigma and hold our heads high, especially when it comes to unjust mental health stigma.

Today, sadly, the troubled behaviors of those who are actively battling mental health concerns are often seen as a choice rather than what they are: symptoms of psychological pain. It is true that psychological distress can present as physical/medical illness. For instance, folks with GI issues and headaches may be experiencing these physical ailments due to high levels of psychological stress. We tend to see this a lot with children—persistent stomach pain every Sunday evening because they are anxious about school Monday morning.

It is hard to believe that in today's information-rich society, many folks are ill-informed or uneducated on mental health problems, creating a rippling effect of embarrassment and shame for individuals with mental health concerns. Ignore those ignoramuses. Hold your head high. You bear no more shame or stigma for issues with stress or mental trauma than you do for a broken leg or a COVID-19 infection. Shame or stigma would not prevent you from getting a broken leg set by a bone doc. Don't let the misplaced stigma of others prevent you from getting mental health help from a head doc!

ANASTASIO

Anastasio was a tall, dark-haired young man whose smile could light up a room. His mother and father immigrated to the United States from southern Italy in the early 1980s. Anastasio's father, Massimo, opened a pizzeria in South Philadelphia while his mother, Vincenza, made her living as a seamstress. She worked out of the family home, making and altering clothes for people in the neighborhood. Anastasio was the oldest of five siblings, attended a Catholic high school for boys, and helped his father at the pizzeria on weekends. His hardworking family were active members of their church.

It was during one of my clinical rotations that I met Anastasio and his parents for the first time. He was referred to the clinic because he was becoming increasingly withdrawn from his family and friends. I also learned that Anastasio had started making claims to his family, such as "I am a prophet who was sent from God to warn humankind about the apocalypse!" He would incessantly quote scripture to his family and talk about the need for repentance to avoid the extinction of humankind.

During our first meeting, I met with Anastasio and his parents. I wanted to ensure that the family was comfortable with me before I asked Anastasio if I could spend some time talking with him one-on-one. They agreed.

At the start of our first session, Anastasio's exchanges with me were appropriate. He did not present as distracted, nor did he display any odd or bizarre behaviors. I could tell he was nervous; he didn't know what to expect. So I spent some time getting to know him. We talked about his likes and dislikes. He shared with me that he really enjoyed making the pizza dough at his father's shop. Anastasio also liked talking with me about his love for soccer. (I learned so much about Italian *calcio* players during my time with Anastasio that I could hold my own in a heated debate with my soccer-obsessed family about the greatest goalkeepers to ever play the game. I'd confidently put my money on Gianluigi Buffon!)

The more time I spent with Anastasio, the more comfortable he grew with me, and the more he trusted me with his feelings and thoughts. He asked me questions about my own religious beliefs, stated the importance of repenting for my sins, and disclosed that he was a prophet sent by God to save humanity.

I realized that he would become so hyper-focused on conveying his message as a prophet that he became disconnected from people. He talked at folks about his mission to save humankind, with no insight or awareness into how his behaviors were affecting others. People in the community felt uneasy around him and avoided him, understandably not wishing to get caught up in a lengthy discussion about God and the salvation of humankind.

These behaviors were episodic and often followed by periods of severe depression, with no talk of his prophecy or compulsion to save the world.

With Anastasio's permission, I met with his parents to discuss his treatment plan. My heart went out to Vincenza as she began to sob in my office when she told me how her son had changed. She explained to me how she had lit a candle for Anastasio in church every day over the past year in hopes that her prayers would help him. Vincenza further explained that she had worried that her son's odd behavior and seeming mental instability would somehow be perceived as a failure by her and her husband. She explained that people within their community had started to look at them differently because of Anastasio's behaviors. They felt judged and alienated because their son was suffering in a way that neither they nor the people in their community understood.

As I spent more time with Anastasio, it became evident that he was struggling with schizoaffective disorder, which is marked by a combination of symptoms associated with schizophrenia-like delusions followed by periods of deep depression or mania. In Anastasio's case, he was experiencing religious delusions rooted in grandiosity because he believed he was a prophet sent to save humankind. When Anastasio's delusions would calm down or dissipate, he would experience depressive symptoms, such as withdrawal from others, excessive sleep, and feelings of over-whelming hopelessness.

Once I had formulated my diagnostic impression, I shared it with Anastasio, knowing that it would be reasonable for him to become irritated, angry, and upset with me. However, I had been seeing him for some time, and he had developed a level of trust with me. I provided him with a safe space where he could share his thoughts and not feel "like he was crazy," judged, or damaged in some way. Anastasio continued in therapy, which was not easy for him. He even began taking psychotropic medication to help decrease his delusions and depressive episodes.

The medications Anastasio was prescribed afforded him the opportunity to talk about things in therapy that were weighing on his mind. I remember him saying, "I feel like a freak. I see how people look at me. They treat me like I'm some kind of nutjob." His eyes were filled with tears. I could hear the pain in his voice. I agreed with Anastasio, validating his feelings. But I thought, *People can be*

People can be such assholes when they don't understand something!

such assholes when they don't understand something! I talked with Anastasio about stigma and how folks with mental health concerns, like schizoaffective disorder, depression, trauma, anxiety —you name it—are often ignorantly judged or dismissed by those who are less educated or less empathetic.

It's as if individuals with mental health concerns are held to an absurd, non-empathetic standard of combating their challenges with sheer willpower. It evokes the expression "Pull yourself up by your bootstraps!" As though the only thing needed to overcome depression or even schizophrenia is willpower. Would anyone fathom giving that kind of advice to a cancer patient?

Anastasio worked through the grief of feeling broken because of the stigma associated with having schizoaffective disorder. Therapy helped Anastasio learn how to manage his mental health rather than be ashamed of it. His parents, Vincenza and Massimo, even participated in their own therapy to process feelings regarding Anastasio's mental health challenges and how they can move through life with a different version of their son than they had anticipated.

Think of it this way: Many of us have dreams or goals that we hope to achieve in life, like getting married, having a couple of children, a successful career, and a beautiful home. We don't plan on having a child with a terminal illness such as cancer or a chromosomal disorder like Down syndrome, but it happens. We optimistically imagine our kids living healthy and carefree lives, not expecting the fastballs that life can throw their way. That is how it was for Vincenza and Massimo; they never imagined that their son would struggle with a mental health concern.

One issue is that mental illness is not a visible illness.

One issue is that mental illness is not a visible illness. You can't see the effects, like those produced by skin cancer or the facial differences observed in folks with Down syndrome. This makes it that much harder for some people to consider mental issues "real" illnesses. Anastasio and his parents were hesitant and afraid to participate in therapy. It took a lot of courage for them to overcome what I refer to as the *dual-stigma effect*.

The first part of the effect questions how we perceive our own mental health challenges. Does our perspective limit the opportunity for us to reach out for help in the first place? Does what we *think* we know about mental health issues impede our ability to seek treatment?

The best way to illustrate this is to provide an example of what your internal monologue might sound like when asked if you believe you're an appropriate candidate for therapy. Your internal voice responds with *Listen Bucko, you don't need therapy because it's reserved for people who are worse off. You're fine. Therapy is for folks who have gone through something terrifying or are crazy. Pour yourself another glass of wine and shake it off!*

What we're actually doing in this scenario is denying ourselves treatment because of the misperception we have created about mental health concerns. Somehow, we don't make the cut because we are capable of functioning to some degree. So our psychological pain is written off, unacknowledged, and not important enough to care for.

The second part of this dual-stigma concept involves dumping a boatload of shame and judgment into the mix. Let's say you understand that your psyche has turned on you, kind of like Regina George in the movie *Mean Girls*, or Jack Torrance in *The Shining*, and you desire mental health treatment. You want to feel better, like yourself again! But you're worried about what everyone else will think or say about it. Your internal voice (aka the little dictator) starts saying things like *People already suspect that you have a few screws loose, but now they are going to know you are unhinged.*

So what do you do? Suffer in silence. You don't reach out for help. Instead, you hope and pray that this too shall pass and that you will wake up one day feeling like the old you.

This way of thinking causes such a mixed emotional reaction for me. I get angry first, then sad. But unfortunately, I get it. I understand how a strong connection has been formed between mental health concerns and mental "weakness." Many of us have been conditioned to believe that reaching out for mental health treatment somehow correlates to being weak-minded, like we aren't capable of dealing with the cards that life dealt us. Well, excuse me, but the thing is, sometimes we *are* handed a raw deal. And when this happens in our lives, the same rules do not apply. Folding on a bad hand in poker doesn't correlate to the same option in life. With poker, you can fold and quit. That's a horrible option in real life, and one none of us should consider for even a moment.

Sadly, some folks feel that they don't have any other choice. They're so overwhelmed with psychological pain that they believe the only way to find relief is to take their own lives. Suicide is a leading cause of death in the United States.

According to the National Institute of Mental Health,[10] 45,979 deaths by suicide occurred in 2020. That is approximately one death every eleven minutes! And when I learned that suicide was the second leading cause of death in young people ages ten to fourteen and twenty-five to thirty-four, I felt the knot in my stomach pull tight. As a society, we have to collectively work together to stomp out the stigma associated with seeking mental health treatment. Kids ten- to fourteen-years-old are taking their own lives because the older generation—their parents (us!)—have done such a poor job addressing our own mental health that we don't know how to help our children. Let me hop on my soapbox for a minute and share with you how seeking mental health treatment has, throughout my life, been a tremendous help for me. Let me preface this by saying that I participated in therapy long before I ever thought about becoming a psychologist.

> . . . suicide was the second leading cause of death in young people ages ten to fourteen and twenty-five to thirty-four.

A Lifetime of Support with Therapy

I shared a bit with you in earlier chapters about my family and the struggles my parents went through regarding drug and alcohol addiction, domestic violence, and financial problems. My mom also suffered with severe anxiety that would sometimes turn into serious bouts of depression.

My parents separated for good when I was in seventh grade. As a kid, I was well aware that my parents had problems within their marriage. You would think that my first reaction would be one of relief when they told me they were getting divorced. But I wasn't relieved; I was afraid. I knew how much worse life could be when they weren't together.

My parents separated for the first time when I was around four years old. Later, when my dad went to prison for dealing methamphetamines, my mother lost herself. She didn't know who she was without my father. My mother is the poster child for co-dependency, and she went off the deep end. She started drinking with her new beau, Eddie, who was very violent toward me and my mother. I never knew what to expect. One minute we were hitchhiking after my mother's car broke down; the next minute we were wandering the streets.

One evening I found myself in a stranger's home, praying that my mom and Eddie didn't forget about me. I must have been asleep when they dropped me off because when I woke up, I had no idea where I was. Looking around, I felt afraid. I remember having to use the bathroom, but I was too scared to get up from the chair and I urinated on myself.

The aftershock trauma I feel, even decades later, has made a lasting impression on me and has affected how I parent my own children. I never want them to feel unsafe or neglected like I did when I was a kid, so I do everything within my control to ensure that their needs are met. Making sure the refrigerator is full of food, that they have clean clothes that fit them, and that my husband and I are consistent and engaged parents are my main priorities. And if I'm being completely honest, I probably go a little overboard giving into their requests for new basketball sneakers every couple of months—so sue me.

The point in sharing this with you is that, from the time I was very young, I was surrounded by an overwhelming amount of stress and chaos. Naturally, existing in a constant state of high stress made me feel very anxious. Oddly enough, as a young kid, I didn't know how to put into words what I was feeling. Google was not a resource that I could tap into when I was a kid (gee, but I'm not that old!).

But I had one thing going for me, something for which I will be forever grateful: my mother's open-mindedness and belief in mental health intervention. Yes, my mom had her fair share of problems, but one admirable thing about her was her willingness to seek treatment, not only for herself but for me.

I was twelve when my parents divorced, and despite all the chaos throughout their marriage, I thought they were better together, mostly because of the practically homeless life I experienced when I was younger. But this time was different. They were splitting up for good this time. I felt like the world was collapsing in on me, and my mother knew it. She helped me by getting me help.

Mrs. Carabelli

When you attend Catholic schools, you have access to CORA services, which stands for Counseling or Referral Assistance. My mom had no shame, knowing what I was going through, about reaching out to CORA and making sure I had access to a mental health professional with whom I could talk on a weekly basis. What I appreciated most was how she explained the CORA services to me. She said, "Geri-Lynn, I know things have been out of control at home. I called your school and got you hooked up with someone you can talk to about how you're feeling. Her name is Mrs. Carabelli."

My mother presented it to me in a positive way. She didn't make me feel like I was "crazy." She made me feel safe and explained to me that Mrs. Carabelli was someone with whom I could share my feelings. Every Tuesday and Thursday, I was excused from eating lunch with my class so that I could speak with Mrs. Carabelli in the CORA trailer (yes, CORA services were located in a trailer outside the school). At first, I felt kind of weird not staying for lunch with my peers. However, when a couple of my close friends asked where I was going, I simply said, "I'm going to talk with Mrs. Carabelli about my parents' divorce."

Because my mother's perception of therapy was one that had no stigma attached, I too learned how to view it in a positive way. She explained that talking to a trained mental health professional about my feelings was healthy for me. She likened it to going to the doctor for a broken bone. The doctor casts the bone to help it heal, she said, in the same way that a therapist can help heal your feelings and emotions about the divorce. It was brilliant!

I didn't fully appreciate the way she framed it until I was much older and realized the stigma connected to mental health concerns. And because I was so honest and matter-of-fact with my peers about talking to Mrs. Carabelli every Tuesday and Thursday, they didn't ask much about it.

I saw Mrs. Carabelli until I graduated from grade school. We talked about a lot of things, from my parents' divorce and how it made me feel to my personal aspirations and goals in life. Some days I talked with her about other things that were causing me stress, like an upcoming science test or trouble I was having with another girl in my grade. Mrs. Carabelli was very easy to talk with; I never felt judged or made to feel guilty or bad about my emotions, feelings, and thoughts. The CORA trailer was a safe place for me, and Mrs. Carabelli earned my trust and created a comfortable environment for me to share my feelings.

Sister Rosemarie

The first year of high school is a transition for everyone. You are meeting new people, navigating new classes, a new building, new teachers, coaches—it's unfamiliar territory. I felt a bit nervous about what to expect upon entering Nazareth Academy, an all-girls private Catholic high school in the northeast section of Philadelphia. Nazareth had an excellent reputation for selecting the brightest girls from the surrounding Catholic grade schools, and it had been a personal goal of mine, from the time I was in sixth grade, to attend Nazareth Academy.

I think a big part of my desire to go originated with my father. He talked about Nazareth like it was the University of Pennsylvania for girls in northeast Philly. I wanted to make him proud, but at the same time, he demonstrated such faith in my intellect and character by taking it for granted that I could get into Nazareth. He believed in me, which helped me believe in myself.

I got in, but it wasn't easy. I always had very good grades, but Nazareth required that all applicants take an entrance test. Passing the test was a part of the acceptance process, in addition to completing an essay and having excellent grades in the sixth, seventh, and eighth grades. Let me put it this way: I nailed it in two of the three requirements but failed the entrance exam miserably. I was so nervous that I don't even think I read all the questions. I was devastated. There was no way I was going to get in with such a poor performance on the entrance exam. Yet I was not going to take no for an answer. I called Nazareth and asked if I could meet with Sister Rosemarie, the principal.

As I walked up the steps to the building and through the glass doors, I felt like I was going to faint, which happens when I feel extremely nervous or stressed-out. I entered the main office, introduced myself to Cookie (yes, really), the secretary, and shared with her that I had a meeting with Sister Rosemarie.

She said, "Have a seat, hon! I'll let Sister know that you're here."

I smiled and sat down in the waiting area.

A few minutes later, a mature woman with bright blue eyes shining under her dark habit came out and walked toward me.

She said, "You must be Geri-Lynn. Come on back."

With that, I followed her back to her office. She pointed toward a chair and directed me to have a seat. She sat across from me and said, "I'm Sister Rosemarie, the principal here at Nazareth. I understand you wanted to meet with me."

I said, "Thank you for meeting with me, Sister. I wanted to talk with you about my entrance exam score. I know it isn't good, but I really want to come to Nazareth."

She looked at me and said, "Why do you want to come to Nazareth?"

I explained, "I think that Nazareth will help prepare me for college, and I want to be the first person in my family to attend and graduate from college."

She looked at me intently for a moment, cracked a big smile, and said, "Geri-Lynn, I'll give you a chance, but you will have to attend the summer program to improve your math skills."

I could feel my eyes starting to well up. I blurted out, "Thank you so much. Sister! I won't let you down!"

She then rose from her chair as if to let me know our meeting was over. I stood up and smiled at Sister Rosemarie. With that, she walked closer to me, extended her arms, and gave me a huge hug. I was caught off guard by her warmth.

What I didn't know at the time was that my mom had called Sister Rosemarie, before my meeting with her, and told her a little bit about what was going on at home, the divorce, and my father moving out. Sister Rosemarie was already prepared to take a chance on me and allow me to attend Nazareth. But at the time, I had no idea that my mother had talked with her. Had I known, I would have been mortified because I was embarrassed by my parents' behavior and by how they had treated each other and me throughout the divorce process. I didn't want Sister Rosemarie to think badly of me because of my wacky family. I didn't realize it back then, but the fear of judgment I carried regarding my family's drug and alcohol abuse, domestic violence, and all-around struggle to be "normal" (whatever I believed that to be at the time) was connected to stigma.

The fear of being judged and treated as "less than" was because my parents had built a fortress in my head. I still talk with my therapist about feeling less than, not deserving of a seat at the table because of my parents' crimes and misdemeanors, as though the manner in which people perceived them has somehow rubbed off on me, making me damaged goods.

> The way you are treated because of what people think they know about mental health concerns . . . makes a lasting impression on how you see yourself.

Intellectually, I understand that this is a flawed way of thinking. However, stigma has that impact on people, even professional shrinks.

The way you are treated because of what people think they know about mental health concerns, such as addiction or depression, makes a lasting impression on how you see yourself—your self-concept. You see, what is even more screwed up is that stigma impacts not only those who are directly suffering with mental health concerns but also those closest to them. My parents' struggles had a direct impact on me and how I saw myself. We look to our environment, the people around us, to affirm who we are. And when that affirmation is negative or damaging, we internalize it and innately adopt it as part of our identity. Is any of this conscious? No, not in the moment. We usually become aware of it in new relationships that we form in adulthood. For example, I learned how to be very independent because of the experiences I had during my childhood. At a glance, you are probably thinking, *That's a great quality!* However, it definitely has a downside.

Now, as an adult, when I feel overwhelmed, I tend to isolate. I try to shoulder whatever mental burden I am struggling with on my own because as a child, I learned that I could not rely on my parents to comfort or console me. It was not safe to share my feelings with them because they were unable to offer the support I needed to feel better. This reinforced for me that the only person I could depend on was myself. Realizing that she could not give me the support I needed as a child, my mother did give me one very important piece of wisdom—the courage to seek mental health treatment when I felt stressed or overwhelmed. Because of the positive experience I had with Mrs. Carabelli in grade school, I sought out counseling services at Nazareth Academy with Mrs. Janotta.

Mrs. Janotta

I was thrilled to have gotten into Nazareth Academy, but at the same time, I always felt like I didn't belong. After all, the actors on the Showtime hit television series *Shameless*, about a dysfunctional family complete with two parents who struggle with addiction and a gaggle of kids who raise themselves, pale in comparison to my family (insert humor as a positive coping strategy here!).

The contention that accompanied my parents' divorce could be likened to the appetizer before the main course. Though it was stressful and sad, it was just the beginning of what lay ahead. My mother's apartment was viewed as a local flophouse where alcohol, drugs, and criminal activity were a requirement for anyone to enter. There were times when the refrigerator was empty, and dinner consisted of what had become our traditional family dinner, a ten-cent pack of ramen noodles.

Of course, I never shared any of this with my friends at Nazareth. I felt ashamed. But rather than having to keep it all in and try to deal with my internal monologue alone, I went to the Counseling and Career Development Office one day during my lunch period.

I asked the secretary if I could speak with one of the counselors about colleges. God forbid I tell the secretary why I was *really* there: "Hi, can I talk to one of the counselors about how incredibly overwhelmed, stressed, and even sad I am because my family is falling apart?" That's not how it works with stigma constantly lurking around in my head and reiterating that I am no good, just like my parents. So I did what any good Catholic would do. I lied.

A few minutes later, a tall, slender woman in her fifties with dark hair and green eyes introduced herself as Mrs. Janotta. Have you ever had the experience of meeting someone and feeling immediate relief, that you could just be yourself? That's how I felt when I met Mrs. Janotta. As soon as she shut the door and I sat down on the chair across from her, I could feel a lump form in my throat. My chin began to tremble, and my eyes filled with tears.

She asked, "What can I do for you, Geri-Lynn?"

And with that simple yet warm introduction, I began to cry. She gave me a minute to calm down and handed me a tissue. I began sharing with her a little bit about my home life and how I felt out of place at Nazareth. She listened intently. Before I knew it, the bell for the next period rang.

Mrs. Janotta said, "Geri-Lynn, please come back and see me. You and I have a lot more in common than you might think."

From that point on, I met with Mrs. Janotta every week. She even shared with me that as a kid, her home life was chaotic too. Through talking with Mrs. Janotta, I gained a sense of hope. She provided a great example for me: you can rise above the challenges you face within your family of origin, carve out your own path, and succeed in life.

> You can rise above the challenges you face within your family of origin, carve out your own path, and succeed in life.

Fast-forward about eight years, and I found myself marching down the aisle to "Pomp and Circumstance" for my college graduation at Cabrini University. I had done it! The support I received from people like Mrs. Carabelli, Mrs. Janotta, and Sister Rosemarie helped me stay on course and accomplish my goals. If it hadn't been for my embracing therapy and utilizing it as a resource or tool when life felt unmanageable, I might have carried the same misconception that many people have about therapy: that it is reserved for people with "real problems" who "really need it."

As a bystander, you would look at me and think that I have it all together. Looks can be deceiving because the truth is that none of us have it all together, certainly not me. That's normal. In fact, it is appropriate. When did modern society get to the point where demonstrating any kind of emotion that isn't "happy" or "positive" is somehow representative of "weakness" or "being dramatic"? Everyone has their own internal struggles that may encompass a range of unhelpful thoughts, from self-doubt to self-loathing.

Dr. Cohen

Once the last assignment has been completed, graduation is typically a happy time for students. For me, the months leading up to my graduation from Cabrini University came with a different kind of stress. I had lived on campus for four years. Though I bounced around from one friend or relative to another during the summer months, I always knew that I would be living on campus nine months out of the year. But after graduation, I knew that I did not have a home, a place to live, and I was scared. I managed to secure a job in radio advertising, which was great, but I needed to figure out where I was going to live.

By this time, my mom's opioid addiction had gotten so bad that she was living on the streets in the notorious Kensington section of Philadelphia. And my relationship with my father was nonexistent at this point in my life.

Turns out, a friend of mine named Tawfiq, "Tuf" for short, had a spare room at his apartment that he offered me after graduation. That helped ease my worries.

Yet, the pressures of being financially independent, mixed with my unrelenting drive to prove to everyone that I could make something of myself in spite of who my parents were, took its toll on me. Not to mention that I was also trying to convince my mother to go to rehab, *and* I was trying to get custody of my eight-year-old half-sister, Dominique, from her father.

With everything going on, I needed to talk with a mental health professional. Not a friend, a *professional*, someone who could provide unbiased, nonjudgmental, and empathetic support. That's when I discovered Dr. Howard Cohen.

I was able to see Dr. Cohen on a weekly basis. His rate was reasonable. I made seeing him a priority, which meant that I had to budget my money wisely. As far as I was concerned, my mental health was worth it.

As with Mrs. Janotta, when I first met Dr. Cohen, I immediately felt comfortable. He was on the short side with a bit of a belly. He wore a loose-fitting polo shirt with khakis and a pair of worn Doc Martens. He had a soft, welcoming voice. I liked his office because he had a tan-colored leather love seat with cotton pillows that I always sat on during our sessions. I would take off my heels, grab a pillow, hold it on my lap, and sit "crisscross-applesauce" on the couch. Dr. Cohen would always sit across from me on a big, comfy chair. The hour would go by so fast.

I would unload the fears, concerns, worries, anger, and sadness I was experiencing onto Dr. Cohen. He would listen and even occasionally slow me down so that he could understand how I was feeling about a particular person or topic. He would interject with bits of feedback that would help me organize my thoughts or see things from a different point of view, which would afford me the opportunity to be kinder to myself.

Dr. Cohen taught me about self-compassion, being gentle, patient, and kind to myself. Because of my own trauma, I defined my value through my accomplishments. My internal monologue, that little dictator that has become a squatter in my psyche, had me convinced that my successes and failures are correlated to my self-worth. Dr. Cohen was one of the first people to help me understand that self-worth isn't all about attaching value to my accomplishments. How I was treating myself and the constant pressure I put on myself to achieve came with a list of side effects that included the inability to relax without feeling guilty. Something as simple as sitting down to watch a movie or take a nap on a Saturday afternoon I could never do. Every minute of every day I had to be doing something "productive." I'd put on a movie while I cleaned the kitchen. Yeah—that was super relaxing.

Aside from feelings of persistent guilt that came by not being productive, there was a toll on my physical body too. When the stress became unbearable, my fainting spells or vasovagal syncope would reemerge. Passing out in the supermarket only to awaken surrounded by a group of strangers is not embarrassing at all. Let's round out this list of side effects with disrupted sleep brought on by the to-do list I put pressure on myself to accomplish by some arbitrary due date.

Moving through life at that pace did a number on my mind and my body. Dr. Cohen's acceptance of me, validation of my feelings, and belief in me helped me begin to understand that giving myself grace and being kind to myself includes respite from the constant work I put into accomplishing my goals. It was a concept that was new to me because I had always existed in a constant state of "go," "perform," and "achieve." He helped me understand that "rest," "refrain," and even "failure" are beneficial components designed to make me stronger—more resilient.

I saw Dr. Cohen for periods of time over a decade. For instance, I might see him every week for six months when I felt really overwhelmed, then stop seeing him for a bit when I felt better and clearer, and then start seeing him again when I felt like I needed support. I saw therapy as a resource that I could tap into when I needed it. And guess what: it worked!

In fact, it worked so well that I shared with Dr. Cohen that I wanted to be a psychologist like him. I wanted the opportunity to help others in the same way that Dr. Cohen helped me.

With a big smile, he said, "I think you should go for it! You would make a great psychologist."

With Dr. Cohen's vote of confidence, I embarked on what would be a nine-year academic journey toward my master's degree in clinical and counseling psychology, followed by my doctoral degree in clinical psychology from Chestnut Hill College.

The Bottom Line: F*$K Stigma

The first hurdle to overcome is learning to say to yourself and truly believe the following: I don't give a flying f*$k what anyone else thinks about me seeking mental health treatment! It's the same thing as getting a tooth filled by the dentist. I wouldn't allow my tooth to rot out of my mouth due to embarrassment or shame of having a cavity, so I'm not going to let my mind (psyche) suffer when therapists exist to help the mind recover in the same way that dentists exist to keep your teeth healthy!

In short, step one is accepting that you can have a mental health concern like depression, high-functioning anxiety, schizoaffective disorder, or aftershock trauma—just look at my story—and seek treatment from a therapist or psychologist no matter how "small" the problem may seem. If it's affecting you and how you feel about yourself, it's worth getting treatment.

The second step is to be courageous enough to ignore other people's misguided judgment around mental health concerns. It all comes back around to accepting and loving yourself enough, despite all your self-perceived "flaws," to get the help you deserve. Remember, you are center stage: the main event. The people who love you will be your backup singers and dancers, and the people who don't understand (or who are feeding the stigma, aka the haters) will be watching you grow from the seats in the nosebleed section! You do you!

SO LET'S REVIEW:

Stigma is that nasty six-letter word that prevents people from reaching for mental health treatment. Why give such a little word so much power?

If your arm was broken, there would be no hesitation in going to the doctor and getting a cast. The same rules apply for your brain—your psyche.

If you are feeling stressed, anxious, depressed, or overwhelmed, go see a mental health professional. Even mental health professionals participate in therapy for themselves.

There is no severity scale that determines whether your struggles or problems are big or bad enough to warrant therapy. If you don't feel like you, that's enough.

You loved your broken arm enough to cast it. Love your psyche enough to speak with a therapist.

CHAPTER SEVEN

What to Expect When Seeking Treatment

WHAT IS THERAPY with a trained mental health professional really like? There's nothing to fear.

A few years back, it seemed as though every pregnant woman was reading the book *What to Expect When You're Expecting*.

This chapter will do much the same: help you understand what to expect when you enter into therapy. Simply knowing what to expect can decrease some of your anxiety and help you take that vital first step. So buckle up, and let's get this ride started.

Here We Go

So! You've finally decided to put your mental health first. You've realized that your psyche should get as much attention as your physical self. Great. I'm proud of you.

It may not seem like a big deal, but making the decision to reach out to a professional for help dealing with those feelings that keep you up at night took courage. We don't typically share these thoughts with anyone, not even those closest to us, out of fear that they'll think we're a few cards short of a full deck. That's fine. *You* are the owner of your thoughts and can choose to share them as you please. Still, making the decision to talk about thoughts that affect your mental health with a trained professional is an admirable choice. Give yourself a pat on the back. You have overcome one of the biggest hurdles to mental health treatment: stigma. But now you're curious to learn what comes next.

What to Expect in Therapy

The first thing to expect is a little bit of paperwork. Just like seeing a primary care provider, you'll fill out forms regarding your contact and insurance information and patient privacy rights, such as how and to what extent others can access information about you. Depending upon the nature of the referral or the reason why you're seeking therapy, a mental health professional may also have you complete a brief questionnaire. For example, if you're seeing a therapist for depression, you might be asked to detail the depressive symptoms you're experiencing. Many times, mental health providers will provide you with these forms ahead of your appointment.

Paperwork aside, it is also important to have a general understanding of the different types of mental health professionals who are able to provide psychotherapy services.

Mental health professionals must be licensed in their respective states in order to conduct therapy. Also, many therapists hold either a master's or doctoral degree in psychology, and with those degrees, they receive certain credentials. For example, I'm a licensed psychologist. After my name, you will see PsyD, which stands for Doctor of Clinical Psychology. You may also see a PhD, which stands for Doctor of Psychology. Both PsyD and PhD signify doctoral-level clinicians. There are also master's level clinicians or therapists who might have the following letters after their names:

- LPC (licensed professional counselor);
- LMFT (licensed marriage and family therapist); and
- LCSW (licensed clinical social worker).

In some fields, such as those involving drug and alcohol, you may see the letters CADC, which stand for Certified Drug and Alcohol Counselor, that is, people qualified to conduct counseling services for individuals with drug and alcohol use disorders.

When seeking mental health treatment, ensure that you're seeing professionals who are *qualified* to deliver therapy services (I know, *duh*, but you would be surprised . . .). Folks who are providing therapy should be licensed in their state of practice to ensure they have been properly trained to conduct therapy. If they aren't licensed and are conducting therapy, they must disclose to the patient that they are working with a licensed mental health professional who is supervising them until they receive their license to practice on their own. You typically observe this with students who are earning their clinical hours toward licensure.

People who are seeking professional therapy should also be weary of "Life Coaches" as "Life Coaches" are not qualified to conduct therapy unless they too are mental health professionals who have earned the appropriate academic degrees (in psychology, sociology, or social work) and are licensed to practice therapy in the state in which you (the patient) reside.

Lastly, psychologists are doctors, but they are not to be confused with psychiatrists, who are medical doctors that specialize in prescribing and managing medications for individuals with mental health concerns.

The First Session

Your first session may take place in person or via telehealth, in which case you'll receive a link in your e-mail that will allow you and your therapist to go face-to-face through the device you are using, like a Zoom meeting. There are also telehealth platforms like BetterHelp and Talkspace that you can access to have sessions with a licensed therapist via a good old-fashioned phone call, or a telehealth session where you can see your therapist on your computer, tablet, or smartphone. Therapy platforms like BetterHelp and Talkspace are purchased via monthly subscriptions.

Of course, some folks prefer telehealth over going to an office because they can participate from the comfort of their own home.

On the other hand, some people prefer an office visit where they can see their mental health provider in person, in an environment that may be less distracting than home. To each their own. Both options are perfectly acceptable, and it really depends on your preference.

During your first meeting, the therapist will go over important safety information with you. This is standard practice. For example, they will ask you to call 911 or go to your local emergency department if you experience a mental health crisis (when you see a therapist in an outpatient setting, like an office, they are not equipped to help you in an active crisis). The therapist will also review the limits of confidentiality with you. For instance, if you disclose that you intend to harm yourself or someone else, the therapist is obligated to share this with the proper authorities to prevent harm to you or another person. To clarify, a therapist will not disclose to your partner if you are having thoughts of infidelity, plagiarized your master's thesis, or if you are questioning your sexual orientation. As long as you do not pose a potential danger to yourself or someone else, what is shared with your therapist stays between you and your therapist.

An example of a mental health crisis is having serious thoughts of hurting yourself or someone else. Your therapist might explain to you what suicidal ideation and suicidal intent are. Suicidal ideation is when you are having thoughts about taking your life because you may feel hopeless or severely overwhelmed. Suicidal intent is when you have thoughtfully constructed a plan of how you intend on taking your own life. Limits of confidentiality can also be broken by your therapist if you disclose during a session you intend to hurt someone or take someone else's life.

An active crisis may also apply to an individual who is experiencing a psychotic break that leaves them disoriented and at high-risk of placing themselves or someone else in a dangerous situation. For instance, I worked with Vincent, a young man in his thirties, who I was seeing at a community mental health clinic. Vincent reported a voice that was telling him to stab his older brother, Joseph, with whom he lived. Vincent was actively psychotic and conveyed to me that the "voices" in his head were telling him to stab Joseph. At that time, Vincent and I had been working together for about four months. He was not compliant with consistently taking his antipsychotic medications, but he was still attending therapy. A big part of why Vincent participated in therapy was because he trusted me and because I didn't treat him like he was "crazy." However, I had to put our therapeutic relationship aside to protect Joseph. Fortunately, Vincent did not want to hurt his brother, but the voices were becoming unbearable for him. It is a therapist's duty to clearly inform patients on the limits of confidentiality to educate them on how the therapist-patient relationship works.

Also at your first visit, a review of the therapist's fees and billing procedures will be shared so that you're clear on your financial responsibility for the service provided. Please keep in mind that some therapists accept insurance and some do not. This should be clearly conveyed to you so that you can make an informed decision as to whether you would like to proceed in therapy with a particular mental health provider.

Once all the safety information, limits of confidentiality, and fees have been reviewed, you find yourself staring at a complete stranger. *Hmmm.*

The therapist may ask, "What brings you into therapy?"

And with that, let the words come. Some folks let it all out. What does that mean? There is no hesitation. You might find yourself walking the therapist through the sequence of events that got you to where you are today. You might even be able to explain how these events have made you feel. Before you know it, the forty-five- to fifty-minute session is coming to a close, and you feel like you have so much more to share, but at the same time you feel like a weight has been lifted from your chest. All the while, you might observe that the therapist is taking diligent notes or actively listening by nodding their head and smiling when appropriate. But the most important thing you might notice is that you feel comfortable and safe sharing your most personal thoughts with them. This is an appropriate response. You are doing great!

Feeling clueless about what to say or how to respond to your therapist's questions during your first visit is also perfectly normal. Heck, even the first handful of times. For some folks, it takes time to warm up to the therapy process. The therapist is a stranger to them. They don't know this person and may not immediately feel compelled to share their most private beliefs with them.

What do these sessions look like? Well, the therapist may work toward getting to know you in a manner that is non-threatening. They might ask what appears to be superficial questions like "What do you like to do for fun? Can you tell me a little bit about your work or school?" By starting a back-and-forth dialogue, you get more comfortable talking about yourself, which can be pretty awkward—I get it! However, as you become more comfortable with the therapist, you will begin to trust them with your feelings. It takes time, and no one should be rushing you, especially your therapist, to share your most personal thoughts and feelings if you aren't quite ready.

It's Not a Perfect Process

Let's look down the road, shall we?

It is imperative that you feel comfortable with your therapist, and feeling comfortable might look different for each of us. For instance, a colleague of mine, Dr. Rivera, was born and raised in Mexico. Naturally, Spanish is her native language. She migrated to the United States to pursue her graduate degree in her midtwenties. Many of the folks that Dr. Rivera sees in therapy are native Spanish speakers who are acculturating to life in the United States. They feel very comfortable with Dr. Rivera because she is able to relate to them in a way that a non-Latino therapist cannot. Connecting with your therapist is the key ingredient, the secret sauce that consists of their ability to make you feel comfortable by accepting you, even the parts of you that you don't like.

Let's say you have been attending therapy for a couple of months and have developed a healthy rapport with your therapist. You feel like they understand you. You can relate to them, and they can relate to you. You trust your therapist, and you don't feel judged, even when you have shared with them some of your dreariest and most menacing thoughts. Nonetheless, you notice that some later sessions leave you mentally drained. You realize that this is different from the feeling of a weight being lifted off your chest that you experienced in previous sessions. You begin to question whether the therapy is working. How *can* it be if you feel so exhausted?

I'm here to tell you that feeling mentally drained or even a little irritable after a therapy session is normal. I know, therapy is supposed to make you feel better. You don't anticipate feeling blah, mentally drained, or even irritable after seeing your therapist. But think about it this way: You are sharing your deepest, darkest, most emotionally evoking feelings with your therapist. The mental energy expended on recounting the memories or events that created a time of turmoil or distress in your life is not meant to be easy. The act of recollecting something that was painful for you may sometimes drag those uncomfortable feelings to the forefront of your mind as opposed to the dark corner in which they have been buried. However, this time you aren't alone. Together, you and your therapist are trying to understand and navigate those feelings. It's not easy, and it shouldn't be.

If you notice that you're feeling emotionally exhausted, share this with your therapist so that you can both dedicate time at the close of each session to practice mindfulness techniques, such as diaphragmatic breathing or being present in the moment, which will help you decompress before going back out into the world.

The key is to keep an open and honest line of communication with your therapist so that you can get the most out of your therapy. Maintaining a forthright dialogue with your therapist will help guide your treatment or indicate that there may be necessary changes. For instance, if you are becoming severely depressed or anxious as a result of your therapy sessions, it might be time to reevaluate your treatment. Remember why you made the decision to enter therapy: to feel better.

So if you notice that you're feeling consistently worse, don't hold it in. Talk with your mental health professional so you can get the kind of help you need.

How Long Should You Go to Therapy?

There is no textbook response for how long someone should attend therapy. Everyone's needs are different. For example, you may be attending therapy because you are feeling anxious about an important event in your life. In my case, after I finished my studies and clinical hours, the next step was to sit for my licensure exam. Fearful of failing the exam and not being able to acquire my license to practice, I was unbearably anxious every time I sat down to study. I was having flashbacks of how miserably I failed the entrance exam to get into Nazareth Academy. I started participating in my own therapy to address the anxiety I was having about the exam. I attended therapy for six months leading up to the exam. After I passed, I took a break from therapy because my anxiety had dissipated after passing the exam!

Thus, the length of time you participate depends on what you're experiencing. I recently ended therapy with a young woman after eighteen months. She had started seeing me after the unexpected death of her fiancé. Together, we concluded that she was feeling much better. She had returned to work, had positive support from her close family and friends, and had been able to move into her own apartment. She utilized therapy to work on her grief. Now don't get me wrong; she is still dealing with the loss of her fiancé. She still experiences feelings of sadness associated with her partner's passing. However, therapy has taught her how to recognize and address her feelings. For now, she is taking a hiatus from therapy, but I am only a phone call away should she want to reengage.

It's a Resource!

We're all busy. Stay-at-home parent, corporate executive, teacher, construction foreman, student, hairstylist, athlete, whatever—we've got plenty to do! Constantly running on life's treadmill is emotionally exhausting. Even though some of us are skilled at juggling multiple balls, we pay a price. That exhaustion leads to bad decision-making, especially when it comes to ourselves and our mental health. In other words, our ignorance about self-care creates a ripple effect in other parts of our lives.

I have been working on being kinder to myself, and therapy has played an integral role in my progress. Yes, therapy! My position as a mental health professional doesn't mean that I don't need help myself! So hear me out before the little dictator in your head propels you into a shame spiral because I mentioned the "T" word.

Therapy is a support, a resource you can tap into, that is designed to help you navigate life when you feel stuck, overwhelmed, or not like yourself. Therapy is not a service that should be ignored until you are at your lowest point of desperation. It is a *support aid* that you can tap into at any time for any reason, no matter how big or small.

Again, I'm a psychologist who provides therapy to other people as a career, and I have a therapist. Look at it this way. I get a full hour to discuss people, places, and things that cause distress in my life with a nonjudgmental, unbiased person who accepts me for who I am and supports me. It doesn't get any better than that.

Consider therapy for yourself—not because you're bonkers but because it can be a useful tool to help you feel better about yourself and better in general.

SO LET'S REVIEW:

Making the decision to participate in mental health treatment is courageous. Congratulations!

Expect a little bit of paperwork, like what you complete for your primary care provider.

Check the professional credentials of your provider. Are they licensed to practice therapy as a counselor, social worker, therapist, or psychologist? And do they have experience in working with people who have mental health concerns similar to yours? Do they accept your insurance? If not, what is their fee?

You can have sessions with your therapist via telehealth or in person depending on how your therapist is set up to see clients.

After a therapy session you might feel energized, like you want to take on the world! This is completely normal. There will also be times when you feel emotionally drained after a session. This too is completely normal. The key is to keep an open line of communication with your provider.

There is no time limit for how long you should participate in therapy. Continually discuss how you are feeling with your therapist and address the best time to terminate treatment collaboratively.

CHAPTER EIGHT

Aftershock in Our "Normal" Lives

IT'S MY HOPE that after reading this book, you've learned that none of us are immune from experiencing some kind of trauma in our lifetime. Being human means experiencing various traumas, but as you've also learned, experiencing something traumatic doesn't mean you'll end up with post-traumatic stress disorder.

PTSD is a diagnosed mental health condition that may result from particularly horrendous circumstances, such as war, sexual assault, a natural disaster, a school shooting, or a home invasion. Victims may later report suffering flashbacks, recurring nightmares, and debilitating anxiety, to name a few symptoms.

Treatment for PTSD requires comprehensive behavioral health intervention that includes intensive therapy and often the support of psychotropic medications.

Nonetheless, it is important to understand the delayed mental health issues that often arise as a result of less extraordinary, *subclinical* types of mental trauma.

All of us will experience life trauma at different times. Divorce, moving to a new city, taking a new job, the illness or death of a loved one, the responsibility of being a parent—these are events and situations that we may all encounter. Yet, as we discussed earlier, it is the very ordinariness of these events that can lead us to overlook the aftershock impact they can have on our lives.

All of us will experience life trauma at different times.

Aftershock speaks to the emotionally distressing and psychologically draining feelings that creep up on us *after* those seemingly conventional experiences. We may feel depressed and anxious weeks or even months after the initial trauma, which may create a sense of confusion, shame, and often intense anxiety as our internal monologue (the little dictator) keeps repeating, *Something is wrong with me. Why do I feel so bad?*

The seeds for PTSD and aftershock are created when, during a time in which we must protect ourselves from the danger of the moment, we push our fears and stress deep down into our subconscious, where it may lie dormant for quite some time. Eventually, it may rage to the surface, often so long after the traumatic event itself that we struggle to connect the problem to the cause.

I'm here to tell you that how you're feeling is completely normal and to let you know that there are things you can do to address these uneasy feelings. You needn't struggle in silence.

So why can't we begin to acknowledge and support what happens to us after we survive the storm of the initial trauma? And why do we feel compelled to minimize situations in our lives that cause delayed negative mental health concerns?

First, recognizing the cause so long after the event is neither intuitive nor a simple diagnostic matter. There are countless situations in life that are highly stressful yet typical. For example, raising kids. Sounds pretty ordinary, right? Maybe not.

People have been procreating for generations, but that does not seem to lessen how emotionally draining it can be. The older folks may have warned us that it wouldn't be easy, but they probably didn't take the time to explain how raising children can feel like walking on a tightrope blindfolded with your feet slathered in petroleum jelly. And as for our kids, we help them try to manage their pain, their joy, their disappointment, and their fears while simultaneously trying to manage our own similar emotions.

Traumatic enough for ya?

So you see, even something as ordinary as raising children can, and likely will, impact your mental health, both when they are still at home and long after.

When they are kids, you might notice that even long after they're feeling better, you are feeling unusually down, on edge, not sleeping well. Even though your child has been able to move on, your psyche is still in overdrive. Having seen your child struggle took a toll on you: aftershock.

And after they're grown, though you might have succeeded in helping your child get through the challenges of childhood, those years of stress did not come without an emotional price, and it may very well be paid in the form of aftershock.

It is vital that you recognize how aftershock may have affected your mental health and that you take steps to lessen the aftershock's ill effects when they do happen.

Don't stick your head in the sand. Take care of your mental health with as much diligence as you care for your physical health. Doing that might include therapy. Remember, therapy is for anyone who is having a difficult time with their mental health. It is not a rare service, reserved only for the most desperate of situations. Don't allow stigma to rear its ugly head and influence that little dictator inside your head.

I hope that by reading this book, you have learned that stigma is the product of miseducation and ignorance. Now, on the other hand, you have the education and knowledge to understand that making your mental health a priority will help to improve your sense of self, which trumps the self-doubt and potential feelings of shame that stigma brings to the table.

You might find yourself at the center of an aftershock storm. It will change how you view the world, yourself, and those around you. But take heart that change isn't always bad.

Surviving challenging times in life doesn't have to mean unpleasant scars. In fact, traumatic events can leave us with marks of wisdom. Noted psychologists Dr. Lawrence G. Tedeschi and Dr. Richard G. Calhoun have taught about PTG—post-traumatic growth—and that we can experience *positive psychological change* as a result of the adversity we've endured. This not only gives meaning to the challenges we have suffered through but actually provides opportunities for extraordinary growth that we would never have been afforded otherwise.

Remember, in life, as in nature, the rain must fall, and it gives life to us all.

Rain is grace;
rain is the sky descending to the earth;
without rain, there would be no life.

—JOHN UPDIKE

SO LET'S REVIEW:

Experiencing traumatic events is all a part of the human experience.

Our responses to the trauma we encounter can be delayed weeks or even months after trauma itself has occurred, hence, aftershock.

Even though we may be struggling with our mental health as the result of a traumatic event, it does not mean that we will meet the diagnostic criteria for PTSD. However, that does not mean that we should ignore how we are feeling.

Reach out for the help and support that you deserve; there is no shame in therapy—go for it!

Always remind yourself that there would be no rainbows without sunshine (the good times) and rain (the bad times).

ACKNOWLEDGMENTS

I WANT TO THANK:

My husband, Greg, for always reminding me what it's all about: family. Your love, genuine support, and infectious laugh help keep me grounded. I love you, Moose!

Gregory, my son, thank you for reminding me what it means to compete hard and stand your ground. Your kind spirit will change the world someday.

Natalee, my daughter, your fierceness and belief in yourself has been an inspiration to witness. I have no doubt that you will take on the world and win!

Dominique, my sister, your energy is undeniably contagious and your "take no shit" attitude is a testament to the kind of strength that cannot be taught. Believe in yourself, Dorkinique—I do.

Sue, my ride or die, when are you going to realize that you are a force to be reckoned with? Jeanette is very proud of you, my dearest friend.

Lee Lee, my littlest sister, graduating college is more than a milestone when your last name is Utter. Enjoy this victory lap, kiddo, because there are many more to come.

Mom, I know you feel a lot of guilt for my crazy childhood—don't. Without you, I wouldn't be me, and I think I'm pretty badass. You did good, kid!

Carol, my mother-in-law, I've always admired your strength. Thank you for giving me Greg.

Kraig, thanks for believing in me, a kid from the wrong side of the tracks. You are the Mickey to my Rocky.

Darcie, thank you for your diligent support through the editing process. You made this experience painless. I am looking forward to working with you on future books.

Steven Seigart from Goldfarb and Associates, it has been refreshing to work with an agent who shares the same tenacity and belief in a project as the author. Your persistence paved the way for opportunity. Thank you.

NOTES

1. Yehuda, Rachel, Nikolaos P. Daskalakis, Linda M. Bierer, Heather N. Bader, Torsten Klengel, Florian Holsboer, and Elisabeth B. Binder. "Holocaust Exposure Induced Inter-generational Effects on FKBP5 Methylation." *Biological Psychiatry* 80, no. 5 (2016): 372–80. https://doi.org/10.1016/j.biopsych.2015.08.005.

2. Dar, Showkat Ahmad, and Dr. P. Sakthivel. "Maslow's Hierarchy of Needs Is Still Relevant in the 21st Century." Research Gate. *Journal of Learning and Educational Policy* 2, no. 05 (2022):1–9 https://www.researchgate.net/publication/362592554_Maslow%27s_Hierarchy_of_Needs_Is_still_Relevant_in_the_21st_Century.

3. Editors, Biography.com. "Sigmund Freud Biography." Biography.com. A&E Networks Television, May 21, 2021. https://www.biography.com/scientists/sigmund-freud.

4. Johnson, Pip. "Good Enough Parenting • Forest for the Trees Perinatal Psychology." Forest for the Trees Perinatal Psychology, August 6, 2021. https://forestpsychology.com.au/good-enough-parenting/#:~:text=Winnicott%20found%20that%20meeting%20the,doing%20so%20boosts%20their%20resilience.

5. "Resilience." American Psychological Association, 2023. https://www.apa.org/topics/resilience.

6. Nortje, Alicia. "Freud's Theory of Humor. - Researchgate." https://positivepsychology.com/defense-mechanisms-in-psychology/. Positive Psychology, April 12, 2021. https://www.researchgate.net/publication/317386267_Freud%27s_theory_of_humor.

7. Ibid.

8. Tedeschi, Richard, and Lawrence Calhoun. "Post-traumatic-Growth: Conceptual Foundations and Empirical Evidence." Research Gate. Psychological Inquiry, November 19, 2009. https://www.researchgate.net/publication/247504165_Tedesch_RG_Calhoun_LGPosttraumatic_growth_conceptual_foundations_and_empirical_evidence_Psychol_Inq_151_1-18.

9. "About Mental Health." Centers for Disease Control and Prevention. Centers for Disease Control and Prevention, June 28, 2021. https://www.cdc.gov/mentalhealth/learn/index.htm.

10. "Suicide." National Institute of Mental Health. U.S. Department of Health and Human Services, 2023. https://www

.nimh.nih.gov/health/statistics/suicide#:~:text=on%20 Suicide%20Prevention.-,Suicide%20is%20a%20Leading% 20Cause%20of%20Death%20in%20the%20United,lives%20 of%20over%2045%2C900%20people.

ABOUT THE AUTHOR

GERI-LYNN UTTER, PSYD, is a clinical psychologist who specializes in working with those struggling with co-occurring mental health concerns, such as trauma and drug addiction. Dr. Utter's motivation for choosing this field was personal; as a child, she frequently witnessed the familial turmoil and violence that arise from such issues. These experiences gave her a rare insight into how our life experiences and the way we see ourselves impact our mental health, both positively and negatively.

Geri-Lynn's experiences have left scars on her soul, which she sees as marks of wisdom that have shaped her understanding of human behavior. She tries to understand what makes people do the things that they do, and this curiosity and desire to help others further drove her to pursue a career as a psychologist.

In 2020, Geri-Lynn released her first book, *Mainlining Philly: Survival, Hope, and Resisting Drug Addiction*, which resulted from her desire to share her story and instill hope in others. The book is based on her life experiences and challenges as a result of her parents' struggles with drug and alcohol addiction, severe anxiety, and depression.

Geri-Lynn currently lives in a Philadelphia suburb with her husband and two children. When she is not practicing psychology or writing, she can be found on the soccer field or basketball court cheering for her kiddos.